CAUSATION
AND PREVENTION
OF HUMAN CANCER

46. F.M. Muggia and M. Rozencweig (eds.): *Clinical Evaluation of Antitumor Therapy.* 1987 ISBN 0-89838-803-1
47. F.A. Valeriote and L. Baker (eds.): *Biochemical Modulation of Anticancer Agents.* Experimental and Clinical Approaches. 1986 ISBN 0-89838-827-9
48. B.A. Stoll (ed.): *Pointers to Cancer Prognosis.* 1987 ISBN 0-89838-841-4; Pb. 0-89838-8767
49. K.H. Hollmann and J.M. Verley (eds.): *New Frontiers in Mammary Pathology.* 1986 ISBN 0-89838-852-X
50. D.J. Ruiter, G.J. Fleuren and S.O. Warnaar (eds.): *Application of Monoclonal Antibodies in Tumor Pathology.* 1987 ISBN 0-89838-853-8
51. A.H.G. Paterson and A.W. Lees (eds.): *Fundamental Problems in Breast Cancer.* 1987 ISBN 0-89838-863-5
52. M. Chatel, F. Darcel and J. Pecker (eds.): *Brain Oncology.* 1987 ISBN 0-89838-954-2
53. M.P. Hacker, Y.S. Lazo and T.R. Tritton (eds.): *Organ Directed Toxicities of Anticancer Drugs.* 1988 ISBN 0-89838-356-0
54. M. Nicolini, (ed.): *Platinum and Other Metal Coordination Compounds in Cancer Chemotherapy.* 1988 ISBN 0-89838-358-7
55. J.R. Ryan and L.O. Baker (eds.): *Recent Concepts in Sarcoma Treatment.* 1988 ISBN 0-89838-376-5
56. M.A. Rich, J.C. Hager and D.M. Lopez (eds.): *Breast Cancer: Scientific and Clinical Aspects.* 1988 ISBN 0-89838-387-0
57. B.A. Stoll (ed.): *Women at High Risk to Breast Cancer.* 1989 ISBN 0-89838-416-8
58. M.A. Rich, J.C. Hager and I. Keydar (eds.): *Breast Cancer: Progress in Biology, Clinical Management and Prevention.* 1989 ISBN 0-7923-0507-8
59. P.I. Reed, M. Carboni, B.J. Johnston and S. Guadagni (eds.): *New Trends in Gastric Cancer.* Background and Videosurgery. 1990 ISBN 0-7923-8917-4
60. H.K. Awwad: *Radiation Oncology: Radiobiological and Physiological Perspectives.* The Boundary-Zone btween Clinical Radiotherapy and Fundamental Radiobiology and Physiology. 1990 ISBN 0-7923-0783-6
61. J.L. Evelhoch, W. Negendank, F.A. Valeriote and L.H. Baker (eds.): *Magnetic Resonance in Experimental and Clinical Oncology.* 1990 ISBN 0-7923-0935-9
62. B.A. Stoll (ed.): *Approaches to Breast Cancer Prevention.* (forthcoming) ISBN 0-7923-0995-2
63. M.J. Hill and A. Giacosa (eds.): *Causation and Prevention of Human Cancer.* 1990 ISBN 0-7923-1084-5
64. J.R.W. Masters (ed.): *Human Cancer in Primary Culture.* A Handbook. (forthcoming) ISBN 0-7923-1088-8

ECP Symposium No. 8

CAUSATION AND PREVENTION OF HUMAN CANCER

Proceedings of the 8th Annual Symposium of the European Organization for Cooperation in Cancer Prevention Studies (ECP),
Heidelberg, Germany, April 2–3, 1990.

Editors:

Michael J Hill, DSc, FRCPath.

Chairman ECP Scientific Committee, Brussels, Belgium;
PHLS Centre for Applied Microbiology and Research,
Bacterial Metabolism Research Laboratory,
Salisbury, UK

and **Attilio Giacosa,** MD

Scientific Coordinator, ECP, Belgium, Brussels;
National Institute for Cancer Prevention, Genoa, Italy

KLUWER ACADEMIC PUBLISHERS
DORDRECHT / BOSTON / LONDON

Distributors

---

for the United States and Canada: Kluwer Academic Publishers, PO Box 358, Accord Station,
Hingham, MA 02018-0358, USA
for all other countries: Kluwer Academic Publishers Group, Distribution Center, PO Box 322, 3300
AH Dordrecht, The Netherlands

British Library Cataloguing in Publication Data

European Organization for Cooperation in Cancer Prevention Studies   *Symposium (8th: 1990:*
   Heidelberg, Germany)
   Causation and prevention of human cancer.
   1. Man. Cancer
   I. Title   II. Hill, M.J. (Michael James) *1939 –*   III. Giacosa, A.
   616.994

   ISBN 0-7923-1084-5

Copyright

Published in the United Kingdom by Kluwer Academic Publishers,
PO Box 55, Lancaster, UK.

Kluwer Academic Publishers BV incorporates the publishing programmes of
D. Reidel, Martinus Nijhoff, Dr W. Junk and MTP Press.

Printed in Great Britain by Butler and Tanner Ltd., Frome and London.

CONTENTS

v

FOREWORD

The European Organization for Cooperation in Cancer Prevention Studies (ECP) was established in 1981 to promote collaboration between scientists working in the various European countries on cancer causation and prevention.

In order to achieve this aim, various working groups - to deal with specific cancers or aspects of cancer aetiology, and to explore the opportunities for advances on a cooperative European basis - were established. It was also decided to hold annual symposia to draw general attention to fields in which there seemed to be many opportunities for progress in matters of prevention.

These symposia have been devoted to themes of high priority to cancer prevention: "Tobacco and Cancer" (1983), "Hormones and Sexual Factors in Human Cancer Aetiology" (1984), "Diet and Human Carcinogenesis" (1985), "Concepts and Theories in Carcinogenesis" (1986)," Preventive Strategies for Cancer related to Immune Deficiencies" (1987), "Gastric Carcinogenesis" (1988), and "Breast, Ovarian and Endometrial Cancer: Aetiological and Epidemiological Relationships" (1989).

This volume contains the proceedings of the 1990 ECP symposium held in Heidelberg, FRG, at the Deutsches Krebsforschungszentrum (DKFZ), on April 2-3 on "Causation and Prevention of Human Cancer".

We are indebted to the speakers for their contribution during the symposium and for their prompt submission of manuscripts. We are grateful to the sponsors, SmithKline Diagnostics and Röhm Pharma.

Our special thanks go to Dr M.C. Stanei-Gueur for preparing and typing the camera forms of all manuscripts.

Michael J. HILL

1
INTRODUCTION AND OVERVIEW OF ECP

Michael J Hill
ECP Headquarters, 5 av. R. Vandendriessche, 1150 Brussels, Belgium

WHAT IS ECP ?

ECP is the European organisation for cooperation in Cancer
Prevention studies and was set up to achieve in the field of
cancer prevention what EORTC attempts to do in the field of
cancer treatment.

WHY SET UP ECP ?

Within the European Community cancer causes more than 700000
deaths per annum, and a good proportion of these must be
preventable. The first step in cancer prevention must be
the determination of cancer causation and, although in the
case of lung cancer this has been known for many years, the
causes of the other major cancers in western populations
have still to be determined. Thus there is a need for large
scale epidemiological studies. Within Europe there is a
wide range in the incidence of most human cancers (Table 1).
This range is far wider than that to be seen within any
single European country; it is also very much wider than
that seen within the United States. Thus, for the planning
of multi-centre cooperative studies of cancer causation
Europe should provide an almost perfect location.
    It has been estimated that 30-40% of human cancers are
caused by dietary factors, principally cancers of the
digestive tract and the hormone-dependent cancers. This
number should be reduced by appropriate changes in the diet
but the optimum diet for prevention of these cancers has
still to be identified. There is a need, therefore, for
large scale multi-centre studies of the relation between
diet and the risk of cancer at the various sites, and to
determine the nature of the mechanisms of dietary
carcinogenesis that need to be countered.

TABLE 1: Range in mortality within the European Community from cancer at various sites (data from Levi et al. 1989)

	Males				Females			
	Max		Min		Max		Min	
Mouth/pharynx	France	15.6	Greece	1.7	Scotland	1.5	Greece	0.6
Oesophagus	France	13.3	Greece	1.9	Scotland	4.0	Greece	0.6
Stomach	Portugal	29.7	Denmark	12.2	Portugal	14.5	France	5.4
Colon/rectum	Denmark	24.3	Greece	7.7	Ireland	18.7	Greece	6.9
Liver	Spain	9.1	Ireland	0.9	Spain	6.3	Portugal	0.4
Pancreas	Netherlands	9.3	Spain	4.3	Denmark	7.1	Spain	2.4
Lung	Scotland	83.5	Portugal	20.1	Scotland	23.2	Portugal	3.6
Ovary					Denmark	10.8	Spain	2.3
Breast					England	28.2	Spain	13.5
Prostate	Belgium	17.5	Greece	7.3				

There is concern about the possible risk of cancer associated with use of the contraceptive pill or of hormone-replacement therapy. Both of these treatments have been in common usage for less than 20 years and so it is too soon to be able to estimate the magnitude of the risk of those cancers diagnosed late in life. Premenopausal cancers are relatively uncommon and so there is need for large scale epidemiological studies to obtain sufficient numbers of cases to give clues to the magnitude of the cancer risk (if any) as soon as possible.

The risks from tobacco usage, other than those directly associated with the smoking of cigarettes, have received relatively little attention. This is understandable but there is now a percieved risk of lung cancer associated with "passive smoking" and a suspected risk associated with tobacco chewing. This latter is now becoming a source of great concern because of the growing popularity of chewing tobacco amongst children in some European countries. Again, it will be necessary to organise studies of large cohorts of, for example, tobacco-chewing children, in order to obtain clear evidence in the minimum time.

Not only does Europe offer a wide range in incidence of all of the most common cancers, it also has a similarly wide range in dietary patterns, environmental exposures (such as, for example, UV light exposure in the UK or Denmark in comparison with Italy or Spain), and of social attitudes to, for example, contraception or sexual freedom. Europe offers an ideal "laboratory" within which to test or to formulate hypotheses on the causation of human cancers, and it would be more sensible to conduct studies of, for example, the role of diet in human cancer within the European context rather than, as at present, within national borders.

A number of cancers are of importance not because they necessarily have a high prevalence but because of the impact of each individual case. One example is cancer of the ovary in young women. Although the actual number of such cases in any individual country each year is small this is the second commonest site of cancer in premenopausal women. Each case usually results in the death of a young mother and the consequence effect on the rest of family, particularly the young children, left behind can be devastating. Since these cancers are not common studies carried out within national boundaries tend to be small and to give statistically insignificant results. It would clearly be better to carry out studies of such cancers at the European, continent-wide, level rather than within national boundaries.

Intervention anywhere in Europe to prevent, or to reduce the incidence of, cancer at the major sites needs to take account of the realities of the Common Agricultural Policy. For example we need to recognize that the amount of money spent on the whole Europe Against Cancer programme is

3

less than 1% of the subsidy given by the CAP to, farmers to Produce tobacco ! For political reasons the CAP also goes against the advice of most health experts in Europe in promoting butter at the expense of margarine and in generally promoting the consumption of meat and dairy products. This very real conflict between the health lobby and the CAP can only be fought at the European level; national campaigns are likely to have much less impact than they warrant.

For all these reasons a group of European scientists and clinicians decided to set up ECP, to try to take advantage of the unique advantages offered by the European "laboratory" to study the causation and then the prevention of the cancers of importance in Europe and to try to operate in parallel with the work of EORTC in the field of cancer treatment.

ORGANISATION OF ECP

The scientific work is divided into 7 broad areas covered by the Working Groups; three of these are site-specific, namely the colon, the stomach and the breast. Three are directed to causes, namely tobacco, virus and AIDS, and hormones and sexual factors. The final one is devoted to public education, since experience with smoking and lung cancer suggests that finding the cause of a cancer may be much simpler than persuading the general public to take the steps necessary to avoid that cause. Each of the working groups has major research projects and also organises the annual symposia and workshops. The Groups and Group Heads are listed in Table 2. Some of the major projects being carried out by the Groups are discussed in detail elsewhere in this symposium in the presentations by the Heads of Groups and so will not be discussed here.

The overall scientific programme of ECP is monitored by the Scientific Committee. This body includes all of the Heads of Working Groups and a number of distinguished

scientists chosen for their expertise in the various aspects of cancer prevention and to include representatives of all countries of the European Community. The current members are listed in Table 3. The Scientific Committee has a Chairman (me) and also has a Scientific coordinator (Dr A. Giacosa) who coordinates and ensures the smooth running of the work of the groups.

The administrative work of ECP is carried out by the Secretariat, based in Brussels. The whole organisation is ultimately controlled by the ECP Administrative Council, which has six members including the Chairman and the Scientific Coordinator. The overall structure of ECP is illustrated in Table 4.

TABLE 2: The scientific groups in ECP and their current heads.

SCIENTIFIC GROUP	CURRENT HEAD
Colon cancer	Prof. J. Faivre (Dijon, France)
Gastric cancer	Dr P.I. Reed (Slough, U.K.)
Breast cancer	Prof. F. de Waard (Bilthoven, The Netherlands)
AIDS/Virus and cancer	Dr P. Ebbesen (Aarhus, Denmark)
Tobacco and cancer	Dr H. Sancho-Garnier (Villejuif, France)
Hormones/sexual factors and cancer	Dr S. Franceschi (Aviano, Italy)
Public education and cancer	Dr V. Wheelock (Bradford, U.K.)

TABLE 3: The ECP Scientific Committee (as at April, 1990)

Name	Country	Main area of expertise
F de Waard	The Netherlands	Head of breast cancer group
J Faivre	France	Head of colon cancer group
P I Reed	U.K.	Head of gastric cancer group
P Ebbesen	Denmark	Head of AIDS/virus group
S Franceschi	Italy	Head of Hormones/sexual factors group
H Sancho-Garnier	France	Head of tobacco group
V Wheelock	U.K.	Head of public education group
R Preussmann	F.R.G.	Chemical carcinogenesis
J Wahrendorf	F.R.G.	Cancer epidemiology
E Benito	Spain	Colorectal cancer
T Salvador-Llivina	Spain	Public education and cancer
A Trichopoulou	Greece	Nutrition and cancer
L Santi	Italy	All aspects of cancer research
C O'Morain	Ireland	Colorectal cancer
C L West	The Netherlands	Nutrition and cancer
L Cayolla da Motta	Portugal	All aspects
A Burny	Belgium	Viruses and cancer
A Maskens	Belgium	Tobacco/Public education
L Dobrossy	W.H.O.	All aspects
J Esteve	I.A.R.C.	Cancer epidemiology/ statistics
A Giacosa	Italy	Scientific coordinator
M Hill	U.K.	Chairman

TABLE 4: The administrative structure of ECP

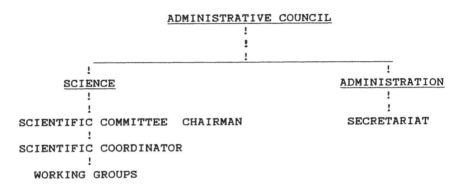

ACTIVITIES OF ECP

In addition to the concerted action research projects carried out by the ECP Working Groups, ECP also organises an annual symposium series and workshops.

TABLE 5: The annual symposia organised by ECP.

YEAR	SUBJECT	LOCATION
1983	Tobacco and human cancer	Brussels
1984*	Hormones and sexual factors in human cancer eatiology	Bruges
1985*	Diet and human cancer	Aarhus
1986*	Concepts and theories in carcinogenesis	Bruges
1987	Preventive strategies for cancers related to immune deficiencies	Brussels
1988*	Gastric carcinogenesis	London
1989	Breast, ovarian and endometrial cancer: epidemiological and aetiological relationships	Bilthoven
1990*	Causation and prevention of human cancer	Heidelberg

* symposium published in the ECP Symposium series.

In the Annual Symposium series the Working Group take turns to choose the topic and to organize the meeting. The symposia are listed in Table 5; the main aim of these symposia has been to present the state-of-the-art in the knowledge of cancer causation and hence prevention of cancer in the field under discussion. One of the annual symposia is going to be organized by the colon group in the near future; this is one of the most active groups in ECP but is

6

the only group that has not yet had one of the symposia.

Each of the working groups has at least one major project in progress, and these go through an evolutionary process outlined in Table 6. All of the projects are reviewed by the Scientific Committee at an early stage and must be approved by that body. Since the Scientific Coordinator is responsible for the coordination of the scientific work of all of the groups, that person is involved in the genesis and development of the projects. The formulation of a project can be simplified by the early organisation of a workshop. This can be used to examine closely a well-defined area of potential research and to prepare for the start of a new project.

TABLE 6: Steps taken in the formulation of an ECP project.
----
1. FORMULATION OF PROJECT <---> SCIENTIFIC COMMITTEE

2. ASSEMBLY OF POTENTIAL COLLABORATORS

3. WORKING PARTY FORMULATES PROTOCOL

4. COLLABORATORS SEEK LOCAL FUNDING

5. ECP SEEKS CENTRAL FUNDING FROM EC

Table 7 lists a number of examples of such workshops organised by the ECP Working Groups. For example, the workshop on "Tobacco and Cancer" in Brussels in 1989 led directly to the formulation of at least three good projects for that Working Group.

One of the major problems with organising multinational concerted-action studies within Europe has been to find funding for the central analyses and coordination of the work. National funding bodies are only willing to fund the analyses of samples from their own country within their own country and have been unwilling to fund analyses from other countries. This, of course, makes nonsense of the concept of multinational collaboration and prevents the clear advantages of central analysis from being realized.

Fortunately, the EC "Europe Against Cancer" programme has been able to fill this gap and to fund the central analyses in a number of ECP projects. The second major problem has been to fund the work in the countries with a low incidence of the cancer of interest, or in those countries where cancer research takes a low priority in comparison with other diseases that are more widespread or more acute. This problem has still to be resolved.

7

TABLE 7: Some of the workshops organised by ECP (other than "progress" workshops)

GROUP	SUBJECT	PLACE	YEAR
Diet	Advice on a healthy diet (with IUNS)	Aarhus	1985
Hormones	Optimisation of influence of ovarian steroid consumption on cancer risk	Munich	1986
Colon	Causation and prevention of colon cancer	Dijon	1987
Tobacco	Tobacco and cancer	Brussels	1988
Public Education	Update or recommendations for healthy eating in relation to cancer	Genova	1990

CONCLUSIONS

ECP has been formed for less than 10 years but has already made a great impression on the cancer research scene, mainly because the need for such a body is so self-evident. In the near future ECP will be ready to publish the results of its first major projects, and will also begin to publish its own journal, the European Journal of Cancer Prevention, in collaboration with Churchill-Livingstone.

8

2

NON-INVASIVE MARKERS OF CARCINOGEN EXPOSURE IN HUMANS

David E G Shuker
International Agency for Research on Cancer, 150 Cours Albert Thomas,
69372 Lyon Cedex 08, France

INTRODUCTION

Human exposure to chemical carcinogens will almost always result in the formation of characteristic adducts with proteins and nucleic acids. This is a consequence of the electrophilic nature of the active metabolites of most carcinogens and the nucleophilic properties of nitrogen atoms present in nucleic acids and sulphur, nitrogen and oxygen atoms in aminoacid residues (1,2). Studies in experimental animals have demonstrated that DNA in target tissue(s) is modified following treatment with many different chemical carcinogens (3). In consequence, there has been much interest in recent years in developing methods to determine the levels of DNA adducts and related damage as an alternative and more relevant measure of human exposure to carcinogens (4). However, in contrast to the situation in experimental animals, only in relatively exceptional cases can DNA from target tissues be obtained from humans and there is, therefore, a need for less invasive methodology which allows access to the same information.

Protein adducts have been investigated as surrogate markers of DNA alkylation. In the case of ethylene oxide, studies have shown that a definite relationship exists between haemoglobin adducts such as N-2-hydroxyethyl-histidine and S-2-hydroxyethylcysteine and DNA adducts such as N-7-(2-hydroxyethyl)guanine (5). 4-Aminobiphenyl, a potent human bladder carcinogen, is present in tobacco smoke and forms an adduct with haemoglobin (6). Aflatoxin B_1 forms adducts with albumin, as well as with liver DNA, and the protein adduct has been used for human biomonitoring (7). From a methodological point of view, the analysis of protein adducts requires only a small sample of blood and quantitation is carried out immunochemically or by gaz chromatography-mass spectometry (GC-MS). It would appear to be the case that the relationship between DNA and protein adduct formation is different for each alkylating agent and the interpretation of the significance of protein adduct levels requires support from experiments in animal models.

Recently developed methodology, which permits a closer approach to target DNA modification than protein adducts, involves the use of lymphocyte DNA. The analysis of adducts in lymphocyte DNA has proved useful in a number of studies including agents such as cis-platin (8), benzo(a)pyrene (9) and N-methyl-N-nitrosourea used in cancer chemotherapy (10). However, the amount of DNA avalaible is normally somewhat limited (a 10 ml blood sample affords 20-30 microgramme DNA depending on the extraction procedure) and application of this dosimeter depends on having very sensitive analytical methodology.

In terms of the amount of adduct for quantitative analysis and ease of collection of samples from human subjects, the use of urinary markers appear to offer certain advantages over the methods described above. It is the object of this summary to discuss the potential of urinary adducts as markers of carcinogen exposure and their role in studies of cancer aetiology and prevention.

URINARY EXCRETION OF DNA ADDUCTS

The repair of modified DNA can take place by a number of mechanisms including excision repair (eg. thymine dimers), depurination through the action of glycosylases (eg. 7-alkylguanines) or dealkylation (eg. O^6-methyl-2'-deoxyguanosine) (11).

Of these repair processes, the most relevant to urinary excretion is that related to glycosylase activity which results in depurination to give the corresponding alkylpurines. However, excision repair can sometimes be of interest as in the case, for example, of 8-hydroxy-2'-deoxyguanosine (8-OHdG). 8-OHdG is the principal product formed from hydroxyl radical attack on DNA. It has been found to be excreted in urine and appears to be related to metabolic rate (12). It is presumably cleaved from DNA by an excision repair pathway and its presence in urine could be indicative of oxidative damage to DNA (since RNA would give the corresponding riboside).

Alkylpurines, resulting from depurination, such as 7-methylguanine (7-MeGua) and 3-Methyladenine (3-MeAde) are almost quantitatively excreted, unchanged, in urine (13,14,15,16). Other alkypurines, including aflatoxin adducts, are known to be excreted in urine, but may be partially metabolized (17). The determination of urinary alkylpurines offers the possibility of an integrated measure of recent (0-48 hr) measure of DNA alkylation in that the urinary product will be derived from adducts in target and non-target tissue.

The measurement of human exposure to aflatoxin B_1 has attracted much attention due to its known animal hepatocarcinogenicity. The development of rapid immunochemical methods (i.e. antibody based affinity columns followed by fluorescence detection) for the measurement of the major aflatoxin-guanine adduct in urine has enabled a large number of human samples to be analysed. Where intake of aflatoxin B_1 could be reliably estimated there did not appear to be a strong correlation between ingestion and excretion of adducts, however, there is almost nothing known about the factors affecting adduct excretion in humans (18). Results from other studies suggest that dietary ingestion of performed aflatoxin adducts (eg. from DNA in meat or vegetables) may be a significant confounding factor (19).

Stable isotope labelling of molecules which are precursors of alkylating species in vivo, is acceptable in human studies particularly during drug development. Recent studies on drugs which are susceptible to N-nitrosation exemplify this approach. Studies in animals have demonstrated that coadministration of deuterium labelled aminopyrine containing a $(CD_3)_2$N-moiety) and sodium nitrite resulted in the dose dependent excretion of deuterium labelled 7-MeGua (20) and 3-MeAde (21). These results clearly establish precursor-product relationships since the incorporation of an intact $-CD_3$ group into the excreted alkylpurine is consistent with intermediate formation of deuterated dimethylnitrosamine and subsequent activation. Although urinary excretion of 7-MeGua could arise from both DNA and RNA methylation this is less likely to be the case for 3-MeAde which is known to be preferentially formed in DNA (with 1-MeAde being formed in RNA) (22). This methodology was applied to human studies on the drug bromhexine, which could form the carcinogenic nitrosamine N-nitroso-N-methylcyclohexylamine (NMCA) after in vivo nitrosation.

Administration of deuterated NMCA to animals resulted in excretion of deuterated 7-MeGua (23). However, in humans administration of deuterated bromhexide did not give rise to detectable levels of deuterated 7-MeGua suggesting that in vivo formation of NMCA did not occur (24,25). However, the presence of large amounts of naturally occurring 7-MeGua (from RNA) interferes with the isotopic analysis at low levels and this sets a practical limit on the sensitivity of the method which is lower than the absolute sensitivity. This problem could, in principle, be reduced by measuring deuterated 3-MeAde, for which there is a much lower interference from the naturally occurring product, and this possibility remains to be exploited .

The apparent absence of 3-MeAde is a naturally occurring methylated base in DNA or RNA lead to the suggestion that measurement of urinary 3-MeAde would be a good marker of DNA methylation (15,22). The development of a sensitive GC-MS procedure for unlabelled 3-MeAde enabled human studies to be carried out and early studies looked very promising (21). Urinary 3-MeAde excretion was approximatively 1000 times lower than 7-MeGua excretion. The production of an antiserum to 3-MeAde (25) allowed the development of immunoaffinity columns which considerably reduced sample preparation time (Friesen et al., manuscript in preparation). Subsequent development of a specific monoclonal antibody to 3-MeAde lead to a rapid completely immunochemical method which was validated by comparison with GC-MS measurements (Prevost et al., submitted for publication).

Studies on human volunteers showed that daily 3-MeAde excretion was very variable, suggesting that there was a dietary component (21). More recent studies on humans eating controlled diets confirmed this observation and showed that more than 90% of urinary 3-MeAde is derived from exogenous sources. However, the relatively easy manipulation of urinary 3-MeAde excretion by dietary means permits model studies to be carried out and preliminary results suggest that human exposure to methylating agents, for example, present in a few cigarettes, can be detected by an increase in urinary 3-MeAde.

It appears that detection of methylation damage by measurement of urinary methylpurines has particular difficulties which are related to ubiquitous nature of biological methylation, which is also unrelated to carcinogenic processes. It is, therefore, much less likely that higher homologues of the alkylpurines will have the same problem and recent work has focussed on methods which permit the identification and quantification of different alkylpurines. Tandem mass spectrometry has been used to identify alkylpurines in urine and there is some evidence of the presence in trace amounts of ethyl- and hydroxyethylguanine in human urine (26). However, this technique is very specialized and expensive and for routine biomonitoring some less sophisticated approach is required. Antibodies are now available which recognize classes of adducts and these can be used to prepare immunoaffinity columns capable of isolating the alkylpurines in one simple step prior to analysis by low resolution GC-MS. One example is 3-benzyladenine (3-BzAde), which may be derived from exposure to benzylating agents such as the oesophageal carcinogen, N-methyl-N-nitrosobenzylamine. Deuterated 3-BzAde is used as an internal standard and 3-BzAde can be quantified by GC-MS following derivatisation (M. Friesen and D. Lin, unpublished observations).

CONCLUSIONS

From the perspectives of cancer causation and prevention, the approaches described above can contribute by enabling the identification of carcinogenic DNA-reactive agents to which humans are exposed and then, by using them as surrogate endpoints, the effectiveness of preventive measures may be evaluated. This overall strategy has been well illustrated by the successful application of the N-nitrosoproline (NPRO) test which allowed the unequivocal demonstration of endogenous nitrosation in humans (27). The determination of DNA damage, as described above, by non-invasive means, may have a great potential for use in human molecular and biochemical epidemiology, in both ecological and prospective studies.

ACKNOWLEGEMENTS

It is a pleasure to acknowledge the continuing support and encouragement of Dr Helmut Bartsch in my work in human biomonitoring. Financial support from a Royal Society European Science Exchange Programme Fellowship, an IARC Visiting Scientist Award and the US National Cancer Institute (Grant No. CA 48473) is gratefully acknowledged.

REFERENCES

1. Miller, E.C. (1978). Some current perspectives on chemical carcinogenesis in humans and experimental animals: Presidential address. Cancer Res, 38, 1479-1496.
2. Singer, B. and Kusmierek, J. T. (1982) Chemical mutagenesis. Ann Rev Biochem, 52, 655-693.
3. Osborne, M. R. (1984) DNA interactions of reactive intermediates derived from carcinogens. In Searle, C.E. (eds), Chemical Carcinogens American Chemical Society, Washington DC, pp. 485-524.
4. Bartsch, H., Hemminki, K. and O'Neill, I.K. (eds) (1988) Methods for detecting DNA damaging agents in humans: Applications in cancer epidemiology and prevention. (IARC Scientific Publication No. 89) Lyon, France: International Agency for Research on Cancer.
5. Fost, U., Marczynski, B., Kasemann, R. and Peter, H. (1989) Determination of 7-(2-hydroxyethyl)guanine with gas chromatography/mass spectrometry as a parameter for genotoxicity of ethylene oxide. Arch Toxicol, Suppl 13, 250-253.
6. Bryant, M. S., Skipper, P.L, Tannenbaum, S.R. and Maclure, M. (1987) Hemoglobin adducts of 4-aminobiphenyl

in smokers and nonsmokers. Cancer Res, 47, 602-608.

7. Wild, C.P., Jiang, Y.-Z., Sabbioni, G., Chapot, B. and Montesano, R. (1990) Evaluation of methods for quantification of aflatoxin-albumin adducts and their application to human exposure assessment. Cancer Res, 50, 245-251.

8. Poirier, M. C., Egorin, M. J., Fichtinger-Schepman, A.M.J., Yuspa, S.H. and Reed, E. (1988) DNA adducts of cisplatin and carboplatin in tissues of cancer patients. In Bartsch H, Hemminki, K. and O'Neill, I.K. (eds), Methods for detection of DNA damaging agents in human: application in cancer epidemiology and prevention (IARC Scientific Publications No. 89) International Agency for Research on Cancer, Lyon, France, pp. 313-320.

9. Perera, F. P., Hemminki, K., Young, T. L., Brenner, D. Kelly, G. and Santella, R.M. (1988) Detection of polycyclic aromatic hydrocarbon-DNA adducts in white blood cells of foundry workers. Cancer Res, 48, 2288-2291.

10. Wild, C.P., Degan, P., Bresil, H., Serres, M., Montesano, R., Gershanovitch, M. and Likhachev, A. (1988) Quantification of 7-methyldeoxyguanosine in peripheral blood cell DNA after exposure to methylating agents. Proc Amer Assoc Cancer Res, 29, 260.

11. Karran, P. and Lindahl, T. (1985) Cellular defence mechanisms against alkylating agents. Cancer Surveys, 4, 585-599.

12. Shigenaga, M.K., Gimeno, C.J. and Ames, B.N. (1989) Urinary 8-hydroxy-2'-deoxyguanosine as a biological marker of in vivo oxidative DNA damage. Proc Natl Acad Sci, 86, 9697-9701.

13. Craddock, V. M. and Magee, P.N. (1967) Effects of administration of the carcinogen dimethylnitrosamine on urinary 7-methylguanine. Biochem J, 104, 435-440.

14. Shuker, D.E.G., Bailey, E., Gorf, S.M., Lamb, J. and Farmer, P.B. (1984) Determination of N-7-($^2H_3$) methylguanine in rat urine by gas chromatography-mass spectrometry following administration of trideutero-methylating agents or precursors. Anal Biochem, 140, 270-275.

15. Hanski, C. and Lawley, P. D. (1985) Urinary excretion of 3-methyladenine and 1-methylnicotinamide by rats following administration of (methyl-14C)-methyl methanesulphonate and comparison with administration of (14C)-methionine or formate. Chem-Biol Interactions, 55, 225-234.

16. Shuker, D.E.G, Bailey, E., Parry, A., Lamb, J. and Farmer, P.B. (1987) The determination of urinary 3-methyladenine in humans as a potential monitor of exposure to methylating agents. Carcinogenesis, 8, 959-962.

17. Shuker, D.E.G. (1989) Nucleic acid-carcinogen adducts in human dosimetry. Arch Toxicol, Suppl 13, 55-65.
18. Groopman, J. D. (1988). Do aflatoxin-DNA adduct measurements in humans provide accurate data for cancer risk assessment? In Bartsch, H., Hemminki, K. and O'Neill, I.K. (eds), Methods for detecting DNA damaging agents in humans: Applications in cancer epidemiology and prevention (IARC Scientific Publication No. 89) International Agency for Research on Cancer, Lyon, France, pp. 55-62.
19. Dragsted, L. O., Bull, I. and Autrup, H. (1989) Substances with affinity to a monoclonal aflatoxin B1 antibody in Danish urine sample. Food Chem Toxicol, 26, 233-242.
20. Farmer, P.B., Shuker, D.E.G. and Bird, I. (1986) DNA and protein adducts as indicators of in vivo methylation by nitrosatable drugs. Carcinogenesis, 7, 49-62.
21. Shuker, D.E.G., Bailey, E. and Farmer, P.B. (1987) Excretion of methylated nucleic acid bases as an indicator of exposure to nitrosatable drugs. In Bartsch, H., O'Neill, I.K. and Schulte-Hermann, R. (eds) The relevance of N-nitroso compounds to human cancer: Exposures and mechanisms (IARC Scientific Publication No. 84) International Agency for Research on Cancer, Lyon, France, pp. 407-410.
22. Lawley, P. D. (1976) Methylation of DNA by carcinogens: some applications of chemical analytical methods. In Montesano,R., Bartsch, H., Tomatis, L. and Davis, W. (eds) Screening tests in chemical carcinogenesis (IARC Scientific Publications No. 12) International Agency for Research on Cancer, Lyon, France, pp. 181-208.
23. Farmer, P.B., Parry, A.J. and Street, B. (1989) Use of deuterium labelling in studies of exposure to carcinogens. In Baillie, T.A. and Jones, J.R. (eds) Synthesis and Applications of Isotopically labelled Compounds (Proceedings of the Third International Symposium on the Synthesis and Applications of Isotopically Labelled Compounds, Innsbruck, Austria, 17-21 July 1988) Elsevier, Amsterdam pp. 375-380.
24. Farmer, P.B., Parry, A., Franke, H. and Schmid, J. (1988) Lack of detectable DNA alkylation for bromhexine in man. Arzneim.-Forsch, 38, 1351-1354.
25. Shuker, D.E.G. and Farmer, P.B. (1988) Urinary excretion of 3-methyladenine in humans as a marker of nucleic acid methylation. In Bartsch, H., Hemminki, K. and O'Neill, I.K. (eds), Methods for detecting DNA damaging agents in humans: Applications in cancer epidemiology and prevention (IARC Scientific Publication No. 89) International Agency for Research on Cancer, Lyon, France, pp. 92-96.
26. Farmer, P.B., Lamb, J. and Lawley, P.D.(1988) Novel uses

of mass spectrometry in studies of adducts of alkylating agents with nucleic acids and proteins. In Bartsch, H., Hemminki, K. and O'Neill, I.K. (eds), Methods for detecting DNA damaging agents in humans: Applications in cancer epidemiology and prevention (IARC Scientific Publication No. 89) International Agency for Research on Cancer, Lyon, France, pp. 347-355.

27. Bartsch, H., Ohshima, H., Pignatelli, B. and Calmels, S. (1989) Human exposure to endogenous N-nitroso compounds: quantitative estimates in subjects at high risk for cancer of the oral cavity, oesophagus, stomach and urinary bladder. Cancer Surveys, 8, 335-362.

3

MEDITERRANEAN DIET AND CANCER

Antonia Trichopoulou, Elias Mossialos and John Skalkides
Ministry of Health and Welfare, Athens School of Public Health,
Department of Nutrition and Biochemistry, L. Alexandras, 196, 11521 Athens,
Greece

INTRODUCTION

Mediterranean diet is a popular but very loose term. Being geographically mediterranean does not necessarily mean that the local dietary profile conforms to the purported mediterranean model, nor is it clear what this model is. It has been common to assume that mediterranean diet is a low fat and particularly low satutared fatty acids diet, but there is now evidence that there is more to this diet than just its fatty acids moiety. Thus Greek diet is high in total fat but low in saturated fatty acids whereas the Southern Italian diet is rich in complex carbohydrates and has a low overall fat content - and yet both regions are characterized by very low incidence rates of coronary heart disease and several form of cancers.

Extensive work has been done on the relation of the mediterranean diet to coronary heart disease, notably by the group of Ancel Keys (1), but there is also evidence that this diet may contribute, in as yet undefined way, to the low occurrence of several forms of cancer and other chronic diseases in this region (2,3).

DATA AND METHODS

In this paper we will review the changes taking place in the mediterranean diet during the recent years and we will try to assess whether the changes in cancer occurrence in a number of mediterranean countries are compatible with the postulated aetiologic links. Four mediterranean countries were considered: Greece, Italy, Portugal and Spain. These are the four European countries that have traditionally been considered as mediterranean. Southern France is of course as mediterranean as any other area, but France as a whole is

more often thought of as an integral part of the more
developed "Western Europe".

The data used were derived mainly from FAO's Food
Balance Sheets (4) and from WHO's World Health Statistic
Annual (5), but other sources were also taken into account.

RESULTS

TABLE 1: Changes of the average food
availability in Greece, Italy, Portugal and
Spain 1961-1985 (in kg per capita per year)

A. Greece

Food groups	1961-65	1971-75	1981-85
Meat	27,0	53,7	68,8
Fish	18,9	14,9	17,6
Milk	129,5	178,4	200,9
Eggs	6,9	10,6	11,3
Cereals	173,2	157,9	143,5
Pulses	8,1	7,1	5,2
Potatoes	33,4	58,0	69,9
Vegetables	104,3	203,2	237,7
Fruits	164,9	170,1	191,8
Sugars	15,9	27,5	34,6
Animal fats	1,9	1,9	2,3
Vegetable oils	17,3	21,7	24,1
Pure ethanol (lt)	5,3	6,1	6,8

B. Italy

Food groups	1961-65	1971-75	1981-85
Meat	34,6	59,9	76,8
Fish	12,6	12,1	13,9
Milk	154,3	203,5	279,6
Eggs	9,4	11,3	11,6
Cereals	178,5	183,9	161,9
Pulses	5,6	4,4	3,4
Potatoes	48,5	39,8	39,6
Vegetables	132,7	150,3	167,6
Fruits	113,2	131,3	124,1
Sugars	26,4	33,0	30,1
Animal fats	4,1	5,9	8,5
Vegetable oils	14,4	20,3	20,9
Pure ethanol (lt)	13,3	13,4	11,7

18

C. Portugal

Food groups	1961-65	1971-75	1981-85
Meat	22,1	38,2	45,5
Fish	55,6	54,6	36,1
Milk	64,6	81,9	98,7
Eggs	3,2	3,6	5,4
Cereals	136,6	136,9	157,6
Pulses	7,0	7,0	5,3
Potatoes	91,6	106,9	96,7
Vegetables	101,4	135,4	132,9
Fruits	78,0	72,5	48,8
Sugars	20,6	27,9	26,7
Animal fats	2,1	2,4	2,8
Vegetable oils	10,1	16,2	16,5
Pure ethanol (lt)	11,1	12,6	18,2

D. Spain

Food groups	1961-65	1971-75	1981-85
Meat	27,2	52,2	70,9
Fish	30,8	37,3	32,2
Milk	92,2	129,9	157,8
Eggs	9,7	13,4	16,3
Cereals	145,8	117,1	114,1
Pulses	7,9	7,6	5,3
Potatoes	112,9	114,2	105,5
Vegetables	136,0	141,5	144,4
Fruits	83,2	121,2	126,0
Sugars	21,6	30,2	30,1
Animal fats	1,7	2,6	2,8
Vegetable oils	15,9	17,3	20,5
Pure ethanol (lt)	9,7	12,0	12,4

Source: Antonia Trichopoulou and Elias Mossialos (6)

Table 1 indicates food availability patterns in the four indicated mediterranean countries during 3 five-year periods spanning a twenty five-year range (6). There are both geographical and time dependent differences that are partly real and partly reflecting variable types of errors in food recording and reporting. There appears to be a decrease in consumption of pulses and, to a lesser extent, cereals and an increase in consumption of eggs, milk products, animal fats and meat. The net results implie a progressive "nothernization" of the mediterranean diet. Further

evidence pointing to the same direction comes from Household
Budget Surveys (7) and from ad hoc studies in several
mediterranean countries (8).

Disease occurrence patterns should be based ideally on
incidence statistics but such statistics are not available
on a country-wide basis in any of the mediterranean
countries. For some diseases, like most cancers, the high
fatality rate allows the use of mortality statistics as
substitutes.

Table 2 shows age standardised (to the world
population) mortality rates, for selected cancers, per
hundred thousand, in Greece, Italy, Portugal and Spain, by
sex, and their ranks among the corresponding rates of 26
European countries (rank 1 indicates the lowest rate). The
cancer sites were chosen as those considered to be more
closely related to diet.

TABLE 2: Age standardised (World) mortality rates from
selected cancers, per hundred thousands, by sex, in
Greece, Italy, Portugal and Spain (1978-1982), and
their ranks among the corresponding rates of 26
European countries (rank 1 indicates the lowest rate).

Cancer		Greece rate	rank	Italy rate	rank	Portugal rate	rank	Spain rate	rank
Oesophagus	M	1,9	3	4,8	17	5,8	20	5,3	19
	F	0,6	6	0,8	11	1,6	21	0,8	14
Stomach	M	12,1	1	22,7	20	29,7	24	19,8	15
	F	6,7	3	10,7	19	14,5	26	9,8	15
Large bowel	M	7,7	1	18,2	12	16,9	9	11,8	5
	F	6,9	1	13,3	11	12,9	10	9,5	6
Breast	M	-	-	-	-	-	-	-	-
	F	14,6	5	19,2	14	15,0	7	13,5	4
Ovary	M	-	-	-	-	-	-	-	-
	F	2,6	3	4,2	6	2,4	2	2,3	1
Prostate	M	7,3	3	10,8	7	13,8	13	12,8	11
	F	-	-	-	-	-	-	-	-

20

DISCUSSION

A comparison among mediterranean countries or between mediterranean and other European countries with respect to cancer mortality rates and food availability patterns may provide some aetiological insights, but valid inferences are hindered by unavoidable errors, frequently systematic, with respect to both cancer registration and food availability recording. Nevertheless it is perhaps suggestive that low consumption of animal fats in the mediterranean countries appears to coincide with the low mortality rates from cancers of the large bowel, breast, ovary and prostate. By contrast, the expected concordance between high consumption of fruits and vegetables and low mortality from oesophageal and stomach cancer is only evident in Greece and not in the other mediterranean countries. This may be due to high intake of salty foods or alcoholic beverages in the latter three countries, or to other more subtle methodologic or substantive reasons.

One way to bypass methodological problems built into international correlations is to assess time trends within particular countries of exposures and disease occurrence indicators. In this instance, however, an assumption has to be made about the component cause-specific disease latency.

Figures 1-6 show time trends during the period 1961-85 of the food groups that have been shown or suspected to be related to the two cancers which are thought of as more strongly related to diet (breast and colorectal). It appears that in the mediterranean countries the availability of meat, animal fats and vegetable oils is increasing (fig. 1,2,3), whereas the availability of cereals and pulses is decreasing, and the availability of vegetables remains stable (with the exception of Greece in which vegetable availability is increasing).

Figures 7 and 8 show secular trends of standardised annual mortality from cancers of the breast (women) and large bowel (both sexes combined).

For breast cancer there has been little overall improvement in medical treatment during the last 20 years and therefore the mortality trends are interpretable in terms of incidence trends. It appears that increase of either energy intake (which is strongly associated with lipid intake) or of intake of lipids themselves (and particularly animal fat) is associated with an increase of the incidence of breast cancer. These data are not discriminatory as to whether it is fat or energy that it is of immediate importance, and do not allow a clear indication as to which is the age at which nutrition is relevant for breast cancer aetiology (perimenarcheal? earlier? later?) but clearly support the notion that

21

CHANGES OVER TIME OF THE AVERAGE DAILY PER CAPITA
AVAILABILITY OF SELECTED FOODS IN GREECE, ITALY, PORTUGAL AND
SPAIN FROM 1961 TO 1985. (Figures 1-6)

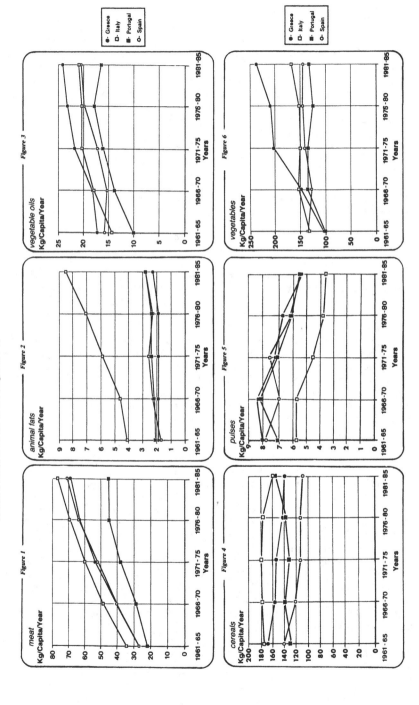

22

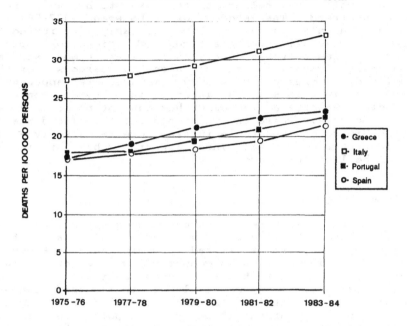

Figure 7 SECULAR TRENDS OF ANNUAL MORTALITY FROM BREAST CANCER IN GREECE, ITALY, PORTUGAL AND SPAIN.

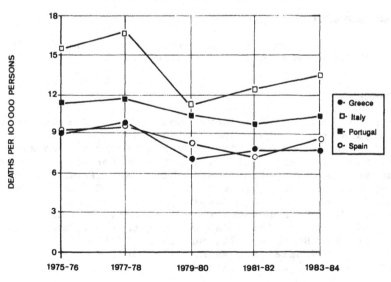

Figure 8 SECULAR TRENDS OF ANNUAL MORTALITY FROM CANCER OF THE LARGE BOWEL IN GREECE, ITALY, PORTUGAL AND SPAIN.

23

nutrition is important in breast cancer causation and that total energy or fat or both are probably implicated.

For colorectal cancer there seems to be an overall increasing trend. The sudden drop between 1977-78 and 1979-80 can only be an artifact, probably attributed to changes in classification practices. The diet link appears likely in view of these data. An increase in meat and fat consumption (vegetable fats may also be hazardous), or the associated increase in energy intake are apparently correlated in time with an increase in the occurrence of colorectal cancer - an increase that can not be compensated by the modest increase in vegetable intake. Incidentally only in Greece did vegetable intake increase markedly - and only in Greece colorectal cancer appears to have stabilized during the last few years.

CONCLUSION

The data presented here are based on geographical patterns and time trends. Since they are ecological (rather than analytical) they are of limited informativeness. However, this limited information is compatible with existing views concerning the nutritional contribution in the multifactorial aetiology of at least two common cancers (breast and colorectal). As such, these data strengthen our convinction that nutrition is an important element in overall health policy objectives and that nutrition policy is an important health priority.

ACKNOWLEDGEMENT

This study was supported, in part, by a grant from Nutra Sweet to the Athens School of Public Health.

REFERENCES

1. Keys ,A. ed. (1980) Seven countries. A multivariate analysis of death and coronary heart diseases. Cambridge, Massachusetts, Harvard University Press.
2. Berrino, F. and Muti, P. (1989) Mediterranean diet and cancer. In the Mediterranean Diet and Food Culture-a Symposium. Edited by Helsing, E. and Trichopoulou, A. Eur J Clin. Nutr., 43, Suppl. 2.
3. Levi, F. , Maisonneuve, P., Filiberti, R., La Vecchia, C. and Boyle, P.(1989) Cancer Incidence and Mortality in Europe. Med Soc Prev, 34, Suppl. 2, 51-584.
4a. (1984) Food Balance Sheets, 1979-1981, Rome.
4b. FAO, personal communication.

5. World Health Organization, World Health Statistics Annual. WHO, Geneva.
6. Trichopoulou, A. and Mòssialos, E. Changing dietary habits in the Mediterranean countries in Europe. Second European Symposium of Cancer Prevention. International Congress Series of Excerpta Medica, Elsevier, Amsterdam, in press.
7. Trichopoulou, A. (1989) Nutrition policy in Greece. In the Mediterranean Diet and Food Culture - a Symposium. Helsing, E. and Trichopoulou A. (eds) Eur J Clin Nutr, 43, Suppl. 2.
8. Ferro Luzzi, A. and Sette, S. (1989) The Mediterranean diet : an attempt to define its present and past composition. In the Mediterranean Diet and Food Culture - a Symposium. Helsing, E. and Trichopoulou, A. (eds) Eur J Clin Nutr, 43, Suppl. 2.

4

EUROPE AGAINST CANCER: 1987–1989 RESULTS AND 1990–1994 PERSPECTIVES

Dr A Vanvossel
Administrator, "Europe against Cancer" programme, DG V, rue de la Loi 200,
B-1049 Brussels, Belgium

The theme of this symposium is "Causation and Prevention of Human Cancer", and as you will see, this is one of the most important fields of action of the "Europe against Cancer" programme. I am therefore pleased to present to you briefly the results of the first action plan and the perspectives for the future.

In recommending the launch of a European programme for the fight against cancer in June 1985 at the European Council in Milan, the Heads of State or Government of the European Community were acting as pioneers. In fact, up until that moment the involvement of the European Community had been limited to only two kinds of actions: firstly, the elaboration of standards of protection for populations against ionising radiation, in the framework of the EURATOM Treaty, and against carcinogenic chemical substances, in the framework of the EEC Treaty, and secondly the prevention of occupational cancers, first of all in the coal and steel industries, in the framework of the ECSC Treaty, and later in all other sectors of activity, in the framework of the EEC Treaty.

It must be stressed, that with these actions, only a small proportion of risk factors were covered, whilst we know that around 75% of cancers are linked to outside factors on which it is possible to act on an individual, national and supranational level.

From 1986 on, with the "Europe against Cancer" programme, the European Community was mobilised in areas other than those where it has a broad competence, as, for example, in the realisation of a genuine Common Market. In addition, the Community has helped to strengthen cooperation between all actors, both public and private, in the fight against cancer in the 12 Member States of the European Community.

Between 1987 and 1989, during the first action plan of

the programme, significant progress was made in the different action areas, these being the prevention of cancer, information and health education, training of health personnel, and medical research.

There were notable results in the area of prevention, particularly in the fight against tobacco, which, as you know, is solely responsible for almost a third of deaths by cancer. Several proposals for Community texts were drawn up by the European Commission and discussed by the European Parliament and the Council of Ministers of the European Community. Certain proposals were even adopted during this first action plan: the Council of Health Ministers adopted on 16 May 1989 a Resolution concerning the banning of smoking in public places. On 13 November 1989 it finally adopted a Community directive requiring the 12 Member States to modify, before 1 January 1993, their legislation on labelling of tobacco products, in order to make smokers more aware of the indisputable risks they are running, by printing clear medical warnings, such as "Smoking causes cancer" or "Smoking causes cardiovascular diseases" on one of the two larger sides of cigarette packets.

In the field of nutrition, the programme played an active role in stimulating and financing epidemiological studies on the link between nutrition and cancer. It is too early to have the results of these studies, but we hope that the work accomplished in these first three years can refine the hypotheses and can be the trigger for important progress in primary prevention in the next 20 years. The programme also initiated a feasibility study for a large prospective nutrition study with several EC countries, which proved that the supranational approach in this field is highly beneficial.

As a final point, I would like to draw your attention to the initiatives in the field of screening. Our Committee of Cancer Experts repeatedly stated that Member States do not take the necessary measures to implement mass screening programmes. We were therefore asked to initiate pilot projects and to link these projects in a network. At present a network of breast screening projects is in operation, comprising six Member States. These pilot projects were selected on the basis of strict criteria fixed by the Committee of Cancer Experts and their work will be evaluated yearly. It should be mentioned that the European programme only covers the launch phase and that the Member States have to provide financial assistance for the running over the following 10 years.

In the near future, similar actions will be undertaken in the field of cervix cancer screening.

I cannot go into detail here, but suffice to mention, several actions were also undertaken in the fight against carcinogenic agents.

As regards information, the main result of the first action plan 1987-1989 was, of course, the realisation in 1989 of the "European Year of Information on Cancer", which mobilised all the Associations and Leagues against cancer, as well as the Ministries of Health and Education, in order to make the general public and young people in schools more aware of the European Code against cancer. In organising the European Year, we had some criticism from the medical world on the effectiveness of such a mass media campaign. It is indeed true that such an initiative is costly (5 million ECUS were spent), and that the evaluation of the action is very difficult. However, we are convinced that such an action is necessary to give political credence. Indeed, with this action we succeeded in mobilising public opinion and consequently the competent authorities of the Member States. I am convinced that this is the reason the new action plan was so quickly and enthusiastically adopted.

The programme was also active in the field of health education. One of the major achievements in this field was the European Conference on Health Education and Cancer Prevention in Schools, which was held in February 1990 in Dublin. During this meeting, recommendations for primary and secondary schools, and for teacher training, were adopted and these recommendations will be discussed at the Council of Education Ministers next May.

In the area of training of health personnel, representatives of all interested parties in the European Community have agreed upon a series of recommendations concerning the training of doctors, dentists and nurses in cancer. As well as this, a hundred doctors and nurses have benefited from training actions in European centres of excellence, in order to perfect their knowledge of screening and treatment of cancer.

Finally, cancer research has been "European-ised" thanks to the encouragement of exchanges of researchers (50 scholarships each year) and the coordination of clinical and fundamental research have even been opened up in the field of improvement of radiotherapy.

Backed up by the satisfying results achieved up until now, the European Commission proposed to the Council and the European Parliament, which as you know are our budgetary authorities, a new five-year action plan which follows the same strategy and axes as the first. The Commission proposed strengthening of the prevention action, the training and health education action and the levelling off of the budget given to information.

In the area of prevention, the European Community will continue its legislative activity in the fight against tobacco, like restriction of tar content of cigarettes, strict reglementation on publicity, banning of oral smokeless tobacco, etc...

Particular emphasis will be given to pilot studies and actions on the links between nutrition and cancer. The large European prospective study mentioned above will be launched and will allow the observation over a number of years of large population samples throughout the European community. Due to the diverse dietary habits in our different countries, it will be possible to determine more precisely the links between certain aspects of diet and cancers of the breast or digestive organs.

In the field of screening, the breast cancer network will be expanded to all countries of the European Community, and at present selection is being made for candidates for the cervix cancer screening. In addition, evaluation studies on the efficiency of colorectal cancer screening will be completed, and small initiatives in the field of prostate cancer detection will be undertaken.

However, the programme does not only want to undertake action in this field, but will also propose legislative measures. Indeed, it is planned to propose to the Council, a recommendation on screening for breast and cervix cancer which will enable us to create a solid base for screening policy in the EEC.

Information and health education actions will continue to make the general public aware of the ten European commandments for cancer prevention. However, it must be stressed that we consider that, notably by organizing the European Year, we have mobilized to a sufficient degree the national associations and leagues, and that these organisms must now take over from the Community the information role. Therefore we will be able to reduce the fraction of the budget to 15% (in the European Year it was 50%).

Based on experience gained in 1988 and 1989, a great many actions on ongoing training for doctors and nurses will receive financial support from the "Europe against Cancer" programme during the next action plan.

The aim is to train trainers and in this way to create a knock-on effect which will harmonize upwards the quality of treatment, screening, etcetera, in the EEC.

For this overall action plan, the Commission requested a budget of 55 million ECUS. (This has to be compared with the budget for tobacco production in the EEC which is 1000 million ECUS).

In November 1989, the Council of Health Ministers adopted the action plan in principle and allowed a budget of 50 million ECUS. The European Parliament gave its opinion on the action plan in March of this year. The opinion is in general favourable, but a certain lack of ambition in the programme is noticed by the Parliament and initiatives in specific fields, like palliative care, quality control of treatment and paediatric oncology are requested. The Parliament also proposes a budget of 80 million ECUS. The

Commission will now propose a modified text to the Council which will take a final decision at the Health Council in May. I am personally convinced that the Council will not change its preliminary decision, and will not take into account the Parliament's opinion. This means that, for the newt five years, we will continue our European Programme with a budget of 50 million ECUS.

Furthermore, the next five years should see the first positive results of concerted actions on medical research, which have been ongoing on since 1987, in the form of pilot projects, notably experimental installations which will enable the treatment of patients by improved radiotherapy. Obviously efforts in coordinating medical research will be pursued and strengthened.

All these actions will only be possible in close cooperation with national and international institutions and organizations like the ECP. However, it is not always easy to combine the initiatives of these organizations with the needs of the programme, and therefore a constant dialogue is necessary. In the past, the programme co-financed, with the ECP, a number of epidemiological studies, which fell within the framework of the programme. We hope that we can continue this collaboration, but in order to do so a mid-term plan is necessary, and we are willing, together with the ECP, to draw up such a plan.

5

PRECANCEROUS LESIONS OF THE COLORECTUM. DESCRIPTIVE EPIDEMIOLOGY AND DIET-RELATED AETIOLOGICAL FACTORS

J Faivre and M C Boutron

Registre des Tumeurs Digestives (Equipe associée INSERM-DGS) Faculté de Médecine, 7 Boulevard Jeanne d'Arc, F-21033 Dijon Cedex, France

ECP Colon Group: D. Beckley (Plymouth), E. Benito (Mallorca), G. Biasco (Bologna), H. Boeing (Heidelberg), M.C. Boutron (Dijon), M. Buset (Brussels), B. Crespon (Paris), R. De Peyer (Geneva), F. Doyon (Paris), J. Faivre (Dijon), A. Giacosa (Genova), M. Hill (Salisbury), A.M. Justum (Caen), H. Kasper (Wursburg), O. Kronborg (Odense), J.L. Lienart (Brussels), W. Matek (Erlangen), C. O'Morain (Dublin), F.M. Nagengast (Nijmegen), P. Pienkowski (Toulouse), J. Pujol (Barcelona), R. Raedsch (Heidelberg), P. Rozen (Tel Aviv), H. Saldanha de Oliveira (Coimbra), M. Thompson (Salisbury), J. Verne (London), M. Wilpart (Brussels), G. Wilson (Edinburgh).

The challenge for researchers addressing the relation between diet and colorectal cancer is to identify the specific dietary determinants of cancer and to quantify their effects. Available data from case-control studies or cohort studies are not sufficient to serve as a basis for strong specific dietary advice. The inconclusive results of the available studies could be explained, at least partly, by the fact that precancerous states have not been taken into account. For this reason there is at the moment a great interest in studies on the relationship between diet and precancerous lesions of the large bowel, i.e. colorectal adenomas.

DESCRIPTIVE EPIDEMIOLOGY OF ADENOMAS

The knowledge of descriptive epidemiologic data on benign and malignant large bowel tumours is of particular importance for understanding the studies focused on the role of diet.

33

1. Do all carcinomas arise on preexisting adenomas ?

Until now only one study has tried to estimate in a direct way the proportion of carcinomas arising from adenomas (1). In his study, Gilbertsen included 18,158 participants with a total of 85,000 person-years. Participants underwent on average 5.4 proctosigmoidoscopies and all polyps found were removed. The author concluded that his policy had reduced the expected incidence of rectal cancer by 85 per cent implicitely stating that at least 85 per cent of rectal cancers arose in adenomas. Unfortunately no conclusion can be drawn from this study because of its methodological problems: no information on subjects lost to follow up, exclusion of the cancer cases discovered at the first screening examination, absence of information on the mode of calculation of "expected" cases, on the frequency of rectal examination or on the characteristics of the diagnosed polyps. Furthermore, this study was limited to rectal cancers and gives no indication on the importance of the adenoma-carcinoma pathway in colon cancers.

In the absence of any way of assessing the importance of the adenoma-carcinoma pathway in cancer formation, the frequency with which remnants of an adenoma are found in invasive carcinomas represents a simple way of estimating what proportion of carcinomas arise from a preexisting adenoma. It has already been well established that the frequency with which a benign tumour is found in continuity with cancer varies with the degree of carcinoma spread (2). In a study of adenomatous remnants in the population-based series of the Côte d'Or, adenomatous tissue was present in 76.5 per cent of the carcinomas limited to the mucosa and submucosa, in 22.7 per cent of those infiltrating the muscularis propria and in 6.2 per cent of those with extramural spread. These data suggest that as cancer spreads through the bowel wall it also expands on the surface of the mucosa and tends to destroy the previous adenoma. Considering that both size and tumour extent are related to the presence of adenomatous tissue, it could be stated that the proportion of colorectal cancers arising in an adenoma is at least equal to 83 per cent which is the proportion of cancers with adenomatous remnants among small cancers less than 2 cm in diameter limited to the mucosa and submucosa. Four factors appeared independently related to the presence of adenomatous tissue within cancers in a multiple regression model. These four variables were by decreasing strength of association: tumour spread, macroscopic type, location and size. Adenomatous remnants were more common in fungating and ulcero-fungating carcinomas than in ulceroinfiltrative and infiltrative carcinomas. In fungating and ulcero-fungating carcinomas, there was a strong relationship between stage of diagnosis and presence of adenomatous tissue. In contrast the association of adenoma remnants and carcinomas was very rare in ulceroinfiltrating and in infiltrating carcinomas whatever the stage of diagnosis. These data support the idea that there could be from the very start two well defined types of cancer, the exophytic one, fungating or ulcero-fungating which would mostly arise in an adenoma, and the endophytic one, ulcero infiltrating or infiltrating, which would be in most cases de novo. This endophytic type represents 40 per cent of all colorectal cancer cases. It has already been emphasized that the distinction might be mainly semantic. Intramucosal adenomas have been observed and it may well be that even seemingly de novo cancers arise on such intramucosal adenomas. But in that case the preexisting adenoma would have no chance of being detected and removed before the occurrence of malignant change.

The frequency of adenomatous tissue was also related to the location of the carcinoma. Cancers in the right colon displayed adenomatous remnants less frequently than those in the left colon or in the rectum for all stages of diagnosis. Our data suggest that although both the adenoma-carcinoma and the de novo pathways occur, their relative importance may vary along the large bowel. Considering the fungating or ulcero-fungating type cancers, it seems reasonable to estimate that most of them arise on preexisting adenomas, at least in the rectum and in the left colon where repectively 80 and more than 90 per cent of the small tumors displayed adenomatous remnants. In the right colon though, the corresponding proportion was only 55 per cent; although there are few limited cases in the right colon and theses figures are to be considered with caution, it can be estimated that some of the fungating right colon cancers do not arise in a polypoid adenoma.

These two pathways of colorectal carcinogenesis, adenoma-carcinoma sequence and de novo carcinogenesis, could relate to different aetiological factors and it will be interesting to take this into consideration in future studies of the genetic and environmental factors responsible for colorectal cancers. As for screening strategies, it would be necessary to take into account that a precancerous lesion or an early cancer is not always detectable and endoscopically removable polypoid lesion.

2. Risk of malignant changes in adenomas:

Clinical studies underline the high prevalence of adenomas in the areas at high risk of large bowel cancer. In France, systematic investigations on asymptomatic subjects aged 45-70 were performed in eight University Departments to estimate the prevalence of adenomas (3). The prevalence of adenomas increase with age from 7 per cent between 45 and 49 to 19 per cent between 65 and 69. In a sample of the Norway population the prevalence of adenomas in the 50-59 age group was found to be 18 per cent (4). These data can be regarded as minimal estimations of the prevalence of adenomas since an endoscopic examination of the large bowel is not as accurate throughout the colon as an autopsy study. In autopsy studies the prevalence of adenomas in subjects more than 65 years old is above 35 per cent (5,6). Thus the prevalence of adenomas is high compared to cancer incidence and it is likely that only a small proportion of adenomas develop into carcinomas.

Clinical studies have shown that a number of factors are of some importance in the development of carcinoma within an adenoma (7,8). It is well established that the malignant potentiality of adenomas is dependant on the size of the adenoma. In the population-based polyp registry of the Côte d'Or the risk of cancers in adenomas under 1 cm in size was only 0.1 per cent (9). Between 1 and 2 cm the risk increased to 9 per cent and over 2 cm in diameter there was a 28 per cent malignancy rate. Other factors than the size of the adenoma such as adenoma type, location of the adenoma, gross morphological pattern and multiplicity of adenomas might also be predictors of the risk of malignancy. But size has the advantage of being easy to evaluate. Available data allow us to conclude that the risk of becoming malignant is exceptional in adenomas less than 1 cm in diameter. A study based on a sample of the Norway population was designed to evaluate the growth rate of polyps less than 5 mm left in the sigmoid or rectum; patients were re-endoscoped after 2 years (10). At that endoscopy 74 per cent of the 194 polyps were recovered for histological examination, 26 per cent were not recovered and a similar proportion of new polyps were registered. Only 40 per cent of the recovered polyps had increased in size and by no more than 3 mm. It was concluded that adenoma less than 5 mm in diameter have a relatively slow growth pattern. This indicates that there is no major risk in leaving small adenomas for later follow-up. It provides an ideal model to study the factors determining the growth rate of adenomas i.e. the most important step in the carcinogenetic process.

Few studies of the natural history of untreated colonic polyps have been reported. A retrospective review of records from the Mayo Clinic for the period preceding the advent of colonoscopy identified 226 patients with colonic polyps more than 10 mm in diameter in whom periodic radiographic examination of the colon was elected over excisional therapy (11). The mean follow up was 68 months, with a maximum of 229 months. During the follow up period 37 per cent of the polyps increased in size. Actuarial analysis revealed that the risk of diagnosing a cancer at the polyp site was 2.5 per cent at 5 years, 8 per cent at 10 years and 24 per cent

36

at 20 years. The corresponding rates for cancer at any site within the large bowel were 5 per cent, 14 per cent and 35 per cent. Those data support the recommendation for excision of all colonic polyps more than 10 mm in diameter. They also underline the fact that a high proportion of large adenomas may remain benign during life time.

3. The adenoma-carcinoma sequence is a multistep process:

The prevalence of adenomas appeared to be higher in men than in women in autopsy studies as well as in clinical studies (6). The male/female ratio for adenomas is always higher than the male/female ratio for cancers in all age groups, especially in young people. For instance in the Côte d'Or the incidence of large bowel cancer was similar among men and women before the age of 60, whereas there was a slight male predominance in older people (9). For diagnosed adenomas there was a male predominance whatever the age with a sex ratio close to 2 in all age groups. These data suggest that if it is supposed that most carcinomas arise from a preexisting adenoma then the rate of transformation of adenoma to carcinoma must be higher in women than in men at the same age. This higher rate of transformation would be determined by sex-related factors such as for example the reproductive history, in addition to risk factors common to men and women.

In clinical studies the segmental distribution of adenomas within the large bowel was not similar to the site distribution of cancers. Carcinomas were more frequently located in the rectum than were adenomas. For instance in the Erlangen statistics 57 per cent of carcinomas were found in the rectum, while only 29 per cent of the adenomas with the highest risk of malignancy were found in that site (12). It was the opposite for the sigmoid. The distribution of adenomas along the large bowel was similar to the distribution pattern of carcinomas only if tumours of the rectum and sigmoid were considered together as it has been done in many statistics. The low frequency of rectal adenomas has been confirmed by autopsy studies (13). Such data suggest that either the adenoma is a less important pathway in the pathogenesis of rectal cancer, or that more rectal adenomas than colon adenomas grow up to a larger size and become malignant. The latter suggestion is supported by the observation that adenomas are larger in the rectum than in other segments. Several studies have shown that malignant changes or severe atypia were found with a higher frequency in the rectum (7,9).

If autopsy and clinical data agree on the low prevalence of adenomas in the rectum they show different distribution patterns in the colon. In autopsy studies the distribution of adenomas was even throughout the bowel, while in colonoscopy studies most colonic adenomas were situated in the left colon. This discrepancy is mainly related to different age patterns of the populations in the autopsy studies compared to the clinical studies (6). Adenomas, the same as carcinomas, are mainly found in the distal colon in 50-65 year old individuals, whereas they predominate in the right half of the large bowel in the older age group. Another reason for the discrepancy between autopsy and clinical data is the frequently incomplete examination of the colon in colonoscopy studies.

Taking into account epidemiological and histopathological data, in particular those relating the malignant potentiality to the adenoma size, Hill et al. (14) have suggested that the large bowel cancer would be a disease with multifactorial aetiology. According to that hypothesis the factors acting at each step of the adenoma-carcinoma sequence i.e. development of a small adenoma, growth towards a large adenoma, and carcinoma may be different. A promoting factor (e.g. diet) is able to produce a cancer only in initiated cells. Thus large bowel cancer could be modulated at different stages of its development. The inconclusive results from case controls studies could be explained by the fact that precancerous states have not been taken into account.

DIET AND LARGE BOWEL ADENOMAS

1. Analytical studies:

It is surprising that there have been so far only two published studies on the role of diet in the occurrence of colorectal adenomas (15,16).

The first study was carried out on 77 cases and an equal number of controls enrolled in a screening program concerning a population sample of 400 subjects from Norway aged 50-59 (15). Fifthy-five cases had polyps less than 5 mm in diameter and 23 had larger polyps. Diet was estimated by asking each individual to register food consumption during five week-days. The authors tried to avoid recall bias by interviewing the subjects before giving them the results of the endoscopy. The results indicated a higher intake of carbohydrates and fibre for controls and a higher intake of fat for cases. This study was well designed, but had the pitfall of a crude statistical analysis comparing only mean values, without adjustement for confounders, in particular caloric intakes.

The second study, performed in Marseille, was based on 250 cases and 250 controls (16). The intake of polysaccharides and natural sugar was lower among cases than among controls, the risk of colorectal adenomas decreasing

38

linearly with increasing daily consumption. In contrast, sugar added to foods and drinks was observed to have the opposite effect i.e. an increasing risk with increasing consumption. The cases also reported a lower consumption of oil, potatoes, K, Mg, and vitamin B6.

Unfortunately none of those studies took into account the multistage concept of the adenoma-carcinoma sequence. For this reason the ECP colon group engaged a case control study in which cases were taken at the three different steps of the adenoma-carcinoma sequence, i.e. patients with the small adenomas less than 1 cm in diameter, patients with large adenomas and patients with cancers. This programme included a large epidemiological study looking mainly at diet and large bowel tumours (which is in progress in Dijon and Genova) and a smaller study in which data on diet as well as on faecal steroids, cell proliferation kinetics and some serological parameters were collected (which is in progress in Brussels, Coimbra, Dijon, Plymouth and Wurzburg). Some results will be available before the end of 1990.

2. Biological studies on bile acids :

The most consistent data on the relationship between colorectal tumours and diet come indirectly from biochemical studies focused on bile acids. Metabolic epidemiological and histopathological studies in humans, experimental studies in rodents and in vitro studies have provided data relating the faecal bile acid concentration to the risk of large bowel cancer (17). In some of those, a detailed analysis has been conducted of the profile of individual faecal bile acids. The ratio of lithocholic to deoxycholic acids has been shown to be higher in cancer cases than in controls. Regarding that ratio, significant differences could also be observed between the 'large adenoma' group (>5mm) and the 'small adenoma' group (18). Such data suggest that the secondary bile acids, i.e. the lithocholic and the deoxycholic acids, and mainly their ratio, are important in the step of adenoma growth i.e. in cancer promotion. They do not seem to play a role in the formation of small adenomas.

An enzyme, the 7-dehydroxylase, produced by gut bacteria, is responsible for the formation in the colon of both lithocholic acid and deoxycholic acid. There is evidence that the activity of this enzyme is higher in large bowel cancer patients than in controls. The 7-dehydroxylase enzyme has an optimum pH close to 7 (close to the usual colonic pH). The pH-activity profile is sharp and activity is much lower at pH 5.5-6.0. Thus from the bile acid hypothesis point of view, a range of possible dietary intervention mechanisms can be formulated with the aim of either decreasing the concentration of faecal bile acids, or of modifying the lithocholic acid/deoxycholic acid ratio, or of quantitatively decreasing the metabolism of the bile acids.

THE FUTURE : INTERVENTION STUDIES

1. Rationale for intervention studies :

Because of the inconclusive results of the available studies, there is at the moment a great interest in intervention studies. They are justified when there is enough evidence supporting the hypothesis that a given diet might be of benefit, but on the other hand the evidence must not be so strong as to make it unethical to withhold the treatment from the control group. We have seen that there are many dietary factors which lead to plausible mechanistic hypotheses about the role they may play in the development of large bowel cancer. As intervention studies are the most powerful tools in cancer epidemiology to detect small or moderate effects which can be of importance to decrease the incidence of this illness it is appealing to investigate some of the available hypotheses within intervention studies.
    The end point of such studies cannot be invasive cancer itself. They would require a very large number of subjects and an excessively long study period. It is therefore not surprising that most planned or on-going intervention studies are conducted in specific high risk populations, mainly patients with adenomas. Most proposed intervention studies use as the end point the development of new adenomas in populations who initially had a clean bowel following polypectomy. Such studies can only usefully test for factors thought to be involved in the causation of adenomas. Yet it is probably the most interesting aspect to study as very little is known about potential aetiological factors acting on this step of carcinogenesis. Most available results and hypotheses, particularly those on secondary bile acids, concern adenoma growth. So it will be interesting to conduct studies in patients with small adenomas left unremoved in the large intestine.

2. The ECP intervention study :

a) Aims :
   The main aim of the study is to test the efficacy of oral calcium supplementation and of oral dietary fibre supplementation in the prevention of colorectal adenomas. This aim will be achieved through a randomized placebo-controlled clinical trial using a parallel design.

The main hypotheses are:
- oral supplementation with (i) 2 g calcium per day (as 5 gr calcium gluconate) or (ii) dietary fibre (as 3.8 gr ispaghula husk), will reduce in patients with a recent personal history of neoplastic polyps of the large bowel: - the new formation rate of such tumours,
- the growth rate of adenomas less than 5 mm left in situ in the large bowel.

Secondary aims are:
- to assess the impact of the initial polyp location and of the previous history of polypectomy on the efficacy of the treatments
- to measure the effect of the treatments on:
  . the modification of colonic cell proliferation,
  . the changes in stools fatty acid composition,
- to explore the relationship between diet, in particular fat and calcium intakes, and the efficacy of the calcium/fibre supplementation.

The study will also allow:
- to investigate in the placebo subjects the relations between diet and recurrence or growth rate of adenomas,
- to determine the new formation/growth rate of adenomas in the placebo group and according to the location of the initial polyp and the previous history of polypectomy;
- to investigate in a large population the relationship between the baseline colonic cell proliferation and the 3-year polyp formation rate of growth,
- to correlate cell proliferation modifications with the new formation rate or growth of adenomas.

b) <u>Study design</u> :
The proposed study design is a parallel design with three arms, namely calcium, fibre and placebo. An alternative had been discussed, that is a 2x2 factorial design which would have had the advantage of estimating the effect of the combination of the two treatments and of performing a truly double blind trial; it would also have given more power to the study with the same number of participants than in the parallel scheme if there was no negative interaction between calcium and fibre. This alternative was abandoned because it was thought unlikely that a good compliance could be maintained over three years with a daily intake of 5 sachets.

c) <u>Study population</u> :
Subjects will be recruited among patients visiting the gastroenterology, surgery or radiology units which will participate in the study in Belgium, Denmark, France, Germany, Holland, Ireland, Israel, Italy, Portugal, United Kingdom, Spain and Switzerland.

The trial will study two aspects:
- the rate at which patients develop new adenomas, in which all included patients will participate;
- the growth rate of the adenoma left behind, which will involve patients with at least one small ($\leq$ 5mm) sigmoidal or rectal polyp. In these patients one of the sigmoidal or rectal polyps will be left behind for studying the growth rate of adenomas and all other polyps will be removed. It was decided to limit the study of the growth rate of a small adenoma to the sigmoid colon and the rectum because it is a small relatively homogeneous region with respect to the growth rate of adenomas and it is easier to find and remove polyps located there.

* <u>Eligible patients</u> will be :
- aged 40 to 75 at entry,
- with a complete colonoscopic examination of the large bowel at inclusion in the study and a "clean colon" except for the polyp left in,
- patients with at least two polyps or patients with one polyp larger than 5 mm in diameter. At least one of the polyps should be a histologically proven adenoma,
- with a pathological examination of all removed polyps,
- with ability and willingness to follow the study protocol,
- having given their written informed consent.
The study coordinator in each centre will be responsible for ascertaining the subjects'eligibility.

* <u>Non-eligible patients</u> will be patients :
- with any severely debilitating or life threatening disease, including invasive cancer in evolution in any site,
- without a complete examination of the large bowel or without a "clean colon",
- without at least one adenoma within the removed polyps,
- with familial polyposis coli,
- with an inflammatory large bowel disease e.g. ulcerative colitis or Crohn's disease,
- with a personal history of colonic resection,
- with an invasive carcinoma in any of the removed polyps
- with a contra-indication to calcium or fibre:
  . history of kidney stones,
  . hypercalcemia,
  . patients already receiving a calcium and/or vitamin D supplementation which cannot be stopped,
  . patients under digitalin treatment,
  . malabsorption syndrome,
  . patients already receiving a regular course of fibre supplement and/or lactulose and who don't accept to

stop them.

d) Size measurement of the left-in polyp :
The ideal for measuring the polyp would have been the
echo endoscope. However as the technique is not yet
available except for experimental centres, we will use a
measuring probe. The polyp will be measured with a
1mm-scaled probe by the endoscopist on three different
axes, the measurement being taken at a rectangular angle
from the polyp, which is made possible by the special
shape of the probe. A photograph of the polyp with the
measuring probe on its side will also be taken for an
easier comparison with the final colonoscopy.

e) Intervention treatments :
- Calcium supplementation:
It will be achieved with Sandocal$^{(R)}$ (calcium
gluconolactate and carbonate). The dose to be
administred will be 2 g calcium per day by means of 2
sachets to be diluted in a glass of water twice a day.
The subjects will be recommended to drink large
quantities of liquid, at least 1.5 l per day, to reduce
the risk of side effects and to take the supplement
before or with the meals rather than between meals.
- Fibre supplementation:
It will be achieved with Fybogel$^{(R)}$ (ispaghula husk),
3.8 g per day as one sachet orange flavoured effervescent
granules to be diluted in cold water and drunk
immediately. The clinician providing the treatment
should emphasize that the granules must be stirred and
drunk immediately without even allowing time for the
granules to dissolve (because the fibre rapidly
transforms into a gel but the patient should in no case
be told this point).
- Placebo :
Two placebos will be used, one with the appearance of the
calcium supplement i.e. 4 sachets a day and the other as
one sachet similar to the fibre treatment. The placebos
will be composed of sucrose plus the same excipient as
for the verum. One half of the control patients will be
given the fibre placebo and the other half the calcium
placebo.

f) Randomization :
The randomization will be stratified on the centre and on
leaving or not one polyp in situ. It will be balanced
every 6 patients in each stratum; that is to say in every
6 patients, two will be allocated the calcium treatment,
two the fibre treatment, one the calcium placebo and one
the fibre placebo. Boxes containing either calcium, or
calcium placebo, or fibre, or fibre placebo will be

numbered according to a computer established randomization list. Each centre will be given two sets of boxes to stratify on leaving or not a polyp : boxes closed with a white sticker for stratum A patients (no polyp left in) and boxes closed with a green sticker for stratum B patients (polyps left in). In each centre and within each stratum the boxes will be given following the increasing order.

The code of the treatment (verum or placebo) will be kept in the randomization centre (F Doyon, Villejuif, France); in case of suspicion of serious side effect (e.g. kidney stones in patients taking the 4 sachets supplement), the randomization centre can be contacted by fax or phone and if necessary, the code will be broken under the responsibility of F Doyon.

g) <u>Sample size</u> :
The rate at which patients are expected to develop new adenomas was estimated from available follow-up studies. It seemed reasonable to expect a 10 per cent annual rate without intervention. The 3-year rate can then be estimated as $1 - (.9 \times .9 \times .9) = .27$. Including 400 subjects in each group will enable the detection of a 10 per cent difference in the rate between the intervention groups and the control group (error $1 = 0.05$, power = 0.90, two-tailed test).

As for the polyp growth study, considering that although there is a larger rate of increase in size than of new adenoma formation a certain proportion of the polyps left in would not be adenomas, it has been calculated (based on reference data from the study by Hoff et al.) that we will end up with similar figures as for the study of recurrence. This will help emphasize how useful it would be to recruit subjects for the two studies at the same time thus reducing considerably the total cost of the study.

It is hoped that each centre will be able to recruit at least 60 patients (but this is in no case a prerequisite for a centre to participate in this study as the usual recruitment in some centres does not yield such a number of eligible patients). The recruitement phase should not last more than 12 to 18 months.

h) <u>Follow-up pattern</u> :
All randomized patients will be followed up every 6 months for three years (even if they stop their treatment) as the analysis will be performed on all randomized patients.
* After the index colonoscopy, the potentially eligible patients will be asked to attend a consultation within about 2 weeks.

At this consultation:
- blood samples will be obtained to measure calcemia and to store blood in aliquots,
- stool samples will be collected,
- a dietary questionnaire will be administered. As there will most probably be an interaction between the subjects normal intake of fibre, calcium and fats, and the treatment efficiency, it is necessary to estimate dietary intakes, with particular emphasis on calcium, fibre and fat intakes i.e. dairy products, vegetables, fruit, cereals, fat and meat intakes. Subjects will be interviewed in a standard way with a dietary questionnaire adapted to the dietary habits of each country. This instrument is a detailed quantitative and qualitative food history questionnaire. A dietician, who has been especially trained in the coordinating centre in Dijon will apply the questionnaire twice, just after the randomization and at the end of the study. This will also permit to evaluate any change in the diet during the course of the study. Each interview will last for about one and a half hours and the questionnaire will be applied unaware of the allocated supplementation.
- a questionnaire on first degree relatives will be administered preferably just after randomization. It will enquire on cancers, colorectal polyps, heart diseases and diabetes. The aim is to have information on epidemiologically related cancers and heart diseases.

All subjects will be briefly interviewed every six months (when they go to the clinic to get their 6 months supply of drug or placebo) to record side effects and to encourage the subjects to continue the study.

Every year blood will be drawn to measure calcemia.

After one year faecal samples will be collected again.

Three years after randomization a full length colonoscopy will be performed and all polyps will be removed and collected for pathological examination. It is of the greatest importance that the final colonoscopy should be performed in the same way as the index colonoscopy and that a control within 3 months should be performed for the same reasons as at entry. The adenoma left-in will be measured with the measuring probe before removal.
- Biopsies will be taken in the low sigmoid for the cell proliferation analysis,
- stool samples will be collected,
- blood samples will be drawn and stored in aliquots,
- a dietary questionnaire will be administered.

No intermediate full length colonoscopy should be performed as this might greatly impair the comparability between groups. In some centres, a one-year control limited to the polyp left in will be performed when considered necessary by the local ethics committee. It is important that this sigmoidoscopy or rectoscopy should be performed only by a physician participating in the study and the polyp should not be removed unless it has notably changed in size or gross appearance. Any other polyp noticed during that examination should not be removed unless larger than 1 cm in diameter or malignant gross appearance.

REFERENCES

1. Gilbertsen, VA. (1974) Proctosigmoidoscopy and polypectomy in reducing the incidence of rectal cancer. Cancer, 34:936-9.
2. Eide, TJ. (1983) Remnants of adenomas in colorectal carcinomas. Cancer, 51:1866-72.
3. Martin, F, Poynard, T, Ribet, A, et al. (1981) A cooperative study on the detection of colorectal cancer and polyps in France. Cancer Detect Prev, 4:407-15.
4. Hoff, G, Vatn, M, Gjone, E, Larsen, S, Sauar, J. (1985) Epidemiology of polyps in the rectum and sigmoid colon. Scand J Gastroenterol, 20:351-5.
5. Williams, AR, Balasooriya, BD, Day, DW. (1982) Polyps and cancer in the large bowel: a necropsy study in Liverpool. Gut, 23:835-42.
6. Vatn, MH. 1987. Epidemiology of adenomas: autopsy data. In: Faivre, J, Hill, MJ (eds). Causation and prevention of colorectal cancer. Amsterdam, Elsevier, ECP Symposium/4, Intern. Congress series 774, pp 13-27.
7. Morson, BC, Bussey, HJR, Day, DW, Hill, MJ. (1983) Adenomas of large bowel. Cancer Surveys, 2:451-77.
8. Hermanek, P, Fruhmorgen, P, Guggenmoos-Holzmann, I, Altendorf, A, Matek, W. (1983) The malignant potential of colorectal polyps. A new statistical approach. Endoscopy, 15:16-20.
9. Faivre, J, Bataillon, P, Hillon, P, Bedenne, L, Boutron, MC, Klepping, C. (1986) L'apport d'un registre de polypes à un registre de cancers colorectaux. In: Groupe pour l'Epidemiologie et l'enregistrement des cancers dans les pays de langue latine. IARC, Lyon, 149-52.
10. Hoff, G, Foerster, A, Vatn, MH, Sayar, J, Larsen, S. (1986) Epidemiology of polyps in the rectum and colon. Recovery and evaluation of unresected polyps 2 years after detection. Scand J Gastroenterol, 21:853-62.
11. Stryker, SI, Wolff, BG, Culp, CE, Libbe, SD, Ilstrup, DM, Mac Carthy, RI. (1987) Natural history of untreated

colonic polyps. Gastroenterol, 93:1009-13.

12. Matek, W, Hermanek, P, Demling, L. (1986) Is the adenoma-carcinoma sequence contradicted by different location of colorectal adenomas and carcinomas ? Endoscopy, 18:17-18.

13. Clark, JC, Collan, Y, Eide, TJ, et al. (1985) Prevalence of polyps in an autopsy series from areas with varying incidence of large bowel. Int J Cancer, 36:179-86.

14. Hill, MJ, Morson, BC, Bussey, MJR. (1978) Aetiology of adenoma-carcinoma sequence in large bowel. Lancet, i:245-7.

15. Hoff, G, Moen, IE, Trygg, K, et al. (1986) Epidemiology of polyps in the rectum and sigmoid colon. Evaluation of nutritional factors. Scand J Gatroenterol, 21:199-204.

16. Macquart-Moulin, G, Riboli, E, Cornee, J, Kaaks, R, Berthezene, P. (1987) Colorectal polyps and diet: a case-control study in Marseille. Int J Cancer, 40:179-88.

17. Thompson, M, Hill, MJ. (1987) Etiology and mechanisms of carcinogenesis. Diet, luminal factors and colorectal cancer. In: Faivre, J, Hill, MJ (eds) Causation and prevention of colorectal cancer. Amsterdam, Elsevier, ECP symposium/4, Int Congress Series 774: 99-120.

18. Owen, RW, Thompson, MH, Hill, MJ, Wilpart, M, Mainguet, P, Roberfroid, M. (1987) The importance of the ratio of lithocholic to deoxycholic acid in large bowel carcinogenesis. Nutr Cancer, 9:67-71.

6

DIET AND PRECANCEROUS LESIONS OF THE STOMACH

P I Reed
Wexham Park Hospital, Slough, Berks, UK

While the incidence of gastric cancer (GC) has been decreasing world wide for over 30 years and has lost its number one world cancer position last year to lung cancer it is still the commonest cancer in the developing countries and because of its poor prognosis has the highest mortality. It is very common in Eastern Asia, Latin America, Eastern Europe and in Europe there is a North-South and East-West gradient (1). In the UK there is also a marked social class gradient in the disease. Furthermore, migrants from high risk areas, such as Japan, moving to low-risk areas (eg Hawaii & California) will retain the high risk for the disease unless they migrated in childhood or early adult life (2). This would suggest an environmental cause for GC with such factors having their effect early in life.

Lauren (3) described 2 major histological types of GC, the intestinal and diffuse. The diffuse type, evenly divided between the sexes has an incidence which is relatively even in all populations, whereas it is the intestinal type of GC which has been decreasing steadily and it is probable that it is its relationship to environmental factors which accounts for the difference in GC incidence between populations.

Although some putative precursors of diffuse carcinoma have been identified, including abnormal mucin goblets and cyto-architectural distortions, this type of cancer is usually discovered **de novo** and very little is known about its epidemiology and aetiology. However, in the case of the intestinal type of cancer much progress has been made in identifying early cancer and precancerous lesions. There is strong evidence especially from populations at high risk of GC to suggest that gastric carcinogenesis of the intestinal type is a multistage process (fig. 1), probably initiated early in life starting with multifocal chronic atrophic gastritis (CAG), progressing to intestinal metaplasia (IM), to epithelial dysplasia (D) and finally to carcinoma (GC). Correa et al. (4) proposed that the reduction of nitrate (NO_3) to nitrite (NO_2) through the action of nitrate

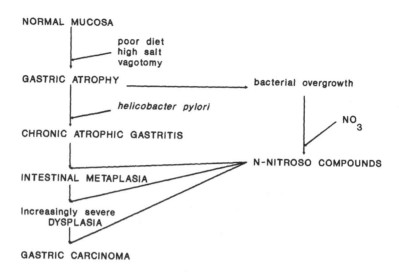

Figure 1. Postulated mechanism for intestinal type gastric cancer aetiology (after Correa et al.)

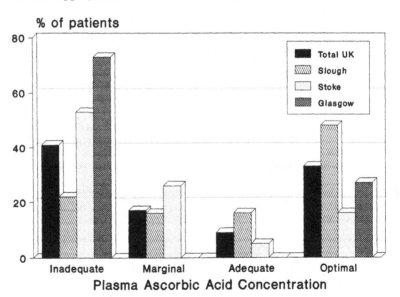

Figure 2. Plasma ascorbic acid status in NC patients.

reducing bacteria in the saliva and in an hypoacidic stomach with the subsequent formation of N-nitroso compounds (NOC) was responsible for the later stage of carcinogenesis.

In recent years several epidemiological studies have made correlations between NO_3 exposure and cancer risk suggesting that a high exogenous exposure increases the risk of cancer (5). This has been contradicted by studies from the U.K. (6-7) showing that the mortality from GC is lowest in areas where NO_3 exposure is the highest, eg in East Anglia in the U.K. However the conclusions drawn from the U.K. studies have been questioned (8-9). Moreover, various factors have to be taken into consideration when relating the exposure to and endogenous formation of NOC, including the nature of the physical source of NO_3, the way in which the NO_3 burden is calculated, the significance of endogenous NO_3 synthesis, the role of dietary or endogenous amines and their potential endogenous nitrosation via chemical interaction, bacterial action or role of stimulated macrophages. All of these may be further influenced by abnormal pathological conditions in the population under investigation. Epidemiological studies often fail to take all these factors into consideration which may account for the contradictions in the literature. It would appear that the diet and dietary sources of NO_3 may be more important than the total nitrate burden, though the latter may be relevant where occasional very high exposures to NO_3 occur. The presence of inhibitors of nitrosation (vitamin C and phenol compounds) occurring concurrently in vegetables will reduce the cancer risk through endogenous NOC formation in low risk populations but with high salivary NO_3 levels.

A recent ECP-Intersalt Collaborative study (10) of 24 hour urinary NO_3 excretion in 5,700 subjects in 48 populations from 28 countries confirmed the very large variations in the intake of nitrate both within and between populations. This was probably due in part to the type of diet, notably vegetables, which generally are the main dietary source of NO_3, and the content of which is related to the level of NO_3 in the soil, being particularly high in volcanic areas. NO_3 excretion was also higher in low income populations, eg in part of Mexico and Eastern Europe but only in the age group 20-29 years, than in more affluent Western populations such as Western Europe and USA.

However, it must be stressed that NO_3 **per se** does not present a cancer risk. It is its action as a precursor to NO_2, via bacterial reduction which can react directly or indirectly (again via bacteria) to produce NOC, known to be potent carcinogens in all 40 experimental animal species so far tested (11,12). It is unlikely that man would be unique as a species and not react to these carcinogens and there is now avalaible a strong body of information that makes it probable that NOC is also carcinogenic in man (4,13-16).

51

In vivo N-nitrosation requires a nitrosatable nitrogen source and a nitrosating agent. Nitrosatable amino and amido compounds are widespread in the human diet. In addition, large amounts of nitrosatable compounds are produced daily as a result of normal human metabolism. Furthermore, while it is possible to determine simple volatile and non-volatile compounds in the diet, the lack of knowledge about specific main precursors to potentially relevant gastric carcinogens is an important limiting factor in the understanding of human gastric carcinogenesis. Positive epidemiological studies have emphasised the nutritional status and specific dietary items relative to GC risk, indicating an increased GC risk with the consumption of smoked, cured or salted meats and fish (Iceland, Japan, Norway) (17), lack of refrigeration (Japan) (18), high NO_3 intake (Chile) (19) as well as a protective effect of yellow-green vegetables (Japan) (20), vitamin C or someother factor in fruit (USA) (21) and a high beta-carotene intake (Switzerland, USA) (22), thus indicating an important role for dietary micronutrients in this regard.

The major source of gastric juice NO_2 is the bacterial reduction of NO_3 and this occurs in the oral cavity and the stomach. Although NO_2 has a very short half-life in the normal acidic stomach, resulting in very low NO_2 concentrations this situation does not pertain once the gastric juice pH exceeds 4 when it is much more stable resulting in much higher gastric juice NO_2 concentrations (23).

Also it must be borne in mind that there are important differences in the rate of formation of NOC. The rate of formation of N-nitrosamines, which are stable compounds requiring biological activation to act as carcinogens, is proportional to the square of the NO_2 concentration while that of the N-nitrosamides of N-nitrosoureas, which are labile and act as direct acting carcinogens especially at higher pH, is directly related to the NO_2 concentration (19). Thus at a given NO_2 concentration the rate of formation of N-nitrosamides may be greater than the N-nitrosamines, an important factor especially when the concentrations of the precursors are low.

The Correa hypothesis (fig. 1) (4) of the formation of intestinal type GC is based on the reduction of NO_3 to NO_2, with subsequent formation of NOC ant their effect on intra-cellular DNA in an abnormal gastric mucosa. At least 5 studies investigating this association have been published (5,24-27), all of which have shown a correlation between gastric juice No_2 and/or bacterial overgrowth and with severity of epithelial dysplasia.

In 1985 the ECP-EURONUT intestinal metaplasia (IM) study was initiated, outlined by West et al (28), its aim being to examine the early stages in the development of the intestinal type of GC with special reference to dietary factors. The study was designed to test the hypothesis that there is a significant difference between intestinal metaplasia patients and matched normal controls with respect to the intake of foods, nutrients and toxicants. Within Europe there is a wide range of dietary habits and a 2.5 fold range in the mortality from GC, Greece having the lowest and Poland and Portugal among the highest. For this reason it was felt that Europe offered the ideal environment to test the hypotheses. In the end 6 countries participated in the study (Table 1) - Greece, Italy, Poland, Portugal, the United Kingdom and Yugoslavia. The original aim was to recruit 150 histologically proven cases of IM per country together with two age and sex matched controls per patient, one with an histologically normal gastric mucosa (EC) and the other a community control with no history of upper gastrointestinal disease (NC). In the core study a questionnaire asked questions about current diet and diet at the age of 25 years. This was a detailed structured questionnaire and included the socioeconomic status and lifestyle, history of smoking habit, alcohol consumption and the use of medicines etc. In addition each patient

TABLE 1: Participating countries and coordinators for the ECP Euronut intestinal metaplasia study.

Country	Coordinator
Greece	A. Trichopoulou
Italy	M. Crespi / A. Giacosa
Poland	L. Hryniewiecki
Portugal	M. Sobrinho-Simoes
UK	M.J. Hill
Yugoslavia	A. Kaic-Rak

contributed a 24 hour urine sample which was assayed for NO_3, sodium, potassium and creatinine. The histological sections were also examined for the presence of **helicobacter pylori**. In the U.K. other peripheral studies were carried out in addition to the core studies. Four centres were chosen in the U.K. (Table 2), Glasgow which has a high rate of gastric cancer and other diet related diseases, Stoke with a high rate of gastric cancer and other dust related diseases both of these centres been in the Northern part of the country, and Slough and London in the South of the

53

country both areas with a low incidence of GC and other diet related diseases (Table 2). Every UK subject had blood taken for the assay of vitamins A, C, E and carotene, selenium, antibodies to **helicobacter pylori** and serum pepsinogens I and II. Gastric juice was collected and assayed for pH, NO_3, NO_2, total and bacterial-reducing bacterial counts. The last patients will be recruited to this study in June 1990 and some preliminary results are available both on the core study and the UK peripheral study.

TABLE 2: Participating centres and staff in the U.K. for the ECP Euronut intestinal metaplasia study.

Center	Participants
Wexham Park Hospital	P.I. Reed
Slough, Berks	M.H. Ali
	D.E. Cussens
	B.J. Johnston
Guy's Hospital,	G. Sladen
London	M.I. Filipe
	D.M. Beswick
North Staffordhire Medical	J.B. Elder
Institute	Histopathology staff
Stoke-on-Trent	A.M. Wilson
Stobhill Hospital	J.A.H. Forrest
Glasgow	G.D. Smith
	J.B. Henderson
PHLS	M.J. Hill
Porton Down	C. Caygill
King's College	P.A. Judd
University of London	

We are presenting here the preliminary results on the vitamin status of 81 age and sex matched sets of UK patients (Glasgow 35, Stoke 18, London 4 and Slough 24) (29). The vitamin levels were divided into 4 bands as given in Table 3.

54

TABLE 3: Definition of vitamin levels.

Vitamin	Inadequate	Marginal	Adequate	Optimal
Ascorbic acid micromol/l	< 20	20-35	35-45	> 45
Carotene micromol/l	< 30	30-70	70-120	> 120
Alpha-tocopherol micromol/l	< 15	15-20	20-25	> 25

The plasma ascorbic acid levels for the non-endoscopic controls (NC) are illustrated in fig. 2 where it can be seen that just over 40% of the control patients had inadequate plasma ascorbic acid levels with a trend towards the patients in the Northern centres having lower levels than those in the South. The carotene levels were also low in about 40% of the NC (fig. 3), again with some evidence of a North/South gradient. Except in Stoke (fig. 4) the majority of patients had adequate of optimal plasma levels of alpha-tocopherol. Figure 5 displays the relationship between the histopathological status and the plasma ascorbic acids levels for the UK as a whole where levels are seen to be lower in IM patients than in the NC. If the results from the 24 sets of patients recruited in Slough are examined in a similar way (fig. 6) it is seen that the IM patients are more likely to have inadequate or marginal plasma ascorbic acid levels and for the NCs to have optimal or adequate levels. If the carotene levels are examined in a similar way (fig. 7) it can be seen that for the UK as a whole there is little evidence for a difference between the patient groups, but if the Slough patients are looked at in isolation there is again a tendency for the IM patients to have lower levels (fig. 8).

To date the only information extracted from the dietary questionnaires is on food groups for 46 sets of UK patients and 28 Polish sets (30). There was a tendency for the IM cases in the UK to have lower intakes of fresh fruit, citrus fruit and salads than the NC group (fig. 9) with a similar trend at age 25 (fig. 10). The results in the Polish patients were similar for current diet (fig. 11) but not at age 25 (fig. 12). This is backed up by the blood level information available for the UK patients. It would appear that in both the UK and Poland the intake of fruit, salad and vegetables appears to be a protective factor. Smoking appears to be related to gastric symptoms in general rather than simply to IM. Histological assessments of the gastric

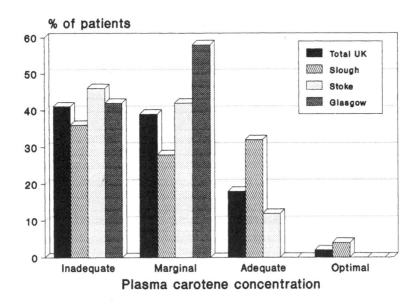

Figure 3: Plasma carotene status in NC patients.

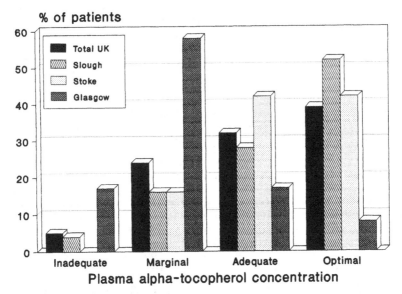

Figure 4: Plasma alpha-trocopherol status in NC patients.

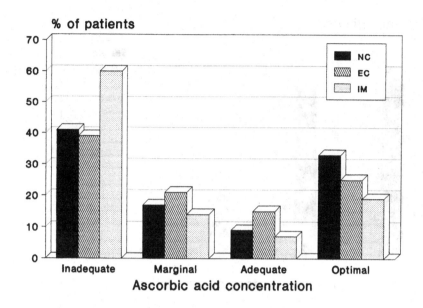

Figure 5: Plasma ascorbic acid status - UK.

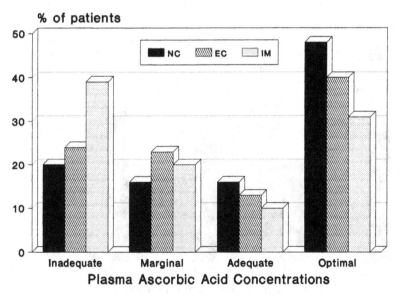

Figure 6: Plasma ascorbic acid status - Slough.

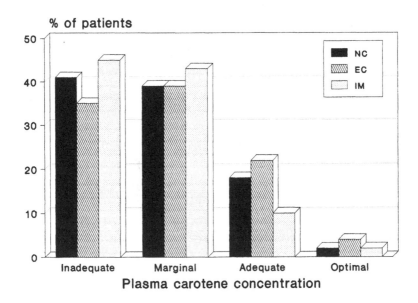

Figure 7: Plasma carotene status - U.K.

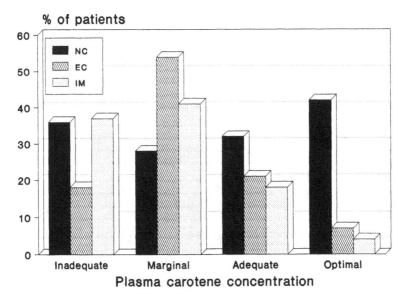

Figure 8: Plasma carotene status - Slough.

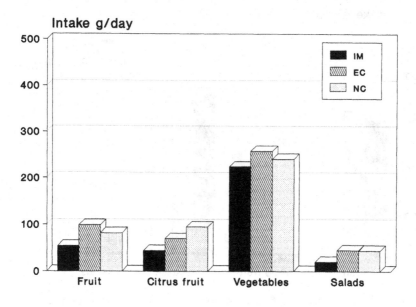

Figure 9: Mean daily food intakes - U.K., current.

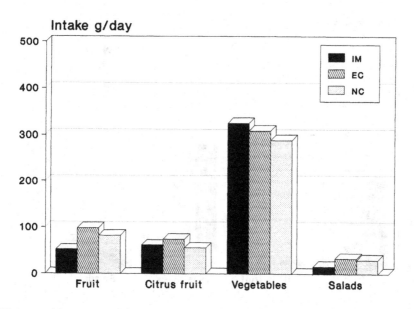

Figure 10: Mean daily food intakes - U.K., age 25.

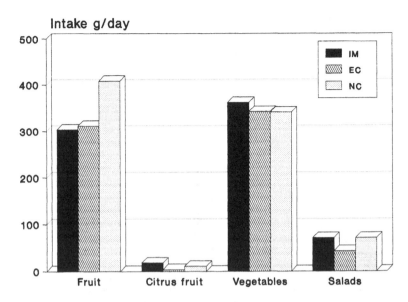

Figure 11: Mean daily food intakes - Poland, current.

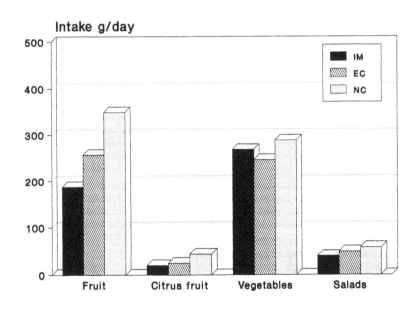

Figure 12: Mean daily food intakes - Poland, age 25.

biopsies revealed that 95% of IM patients were colonised with HP compared to only 6% of endoscopic controls. It is important to remember that all the results described here are preliminary and that many more patients have been recruited to the study than were available for this analysis.

The most helpful way of decreasing the rate of GC further would be by carrying out intervention studies especially in higher risk populations. The few limited intervention trials carried out so far in man have shown encouraging results.

Correa et al. (Personal communication) initiated a pilot study in a high risk area of Colombia (Narino) studying the possible effects of two months administration of vitamins C, E and A independently on the gastric mucosa in subjects with severe chronic gastritis. Twenty matched subjects in each of three active treatment groups were compared with a fourth group given placebo tablets. Although no significant histological changes were observed in the course of such a short study, nevertheless this study did demonstrate good compliance and offered encouragement for carrying out future large-scale intervention trials.

In another study Kyrtopoulos (31) supplemented the diet of a group of Greek trialists with 400 mg daily each of vitamin C and alpha-tocopherol, and demonstrated a significant reduction of mutagenic compounds excreted with the faeces suggesting the presence of endogenously formed mutagens the formation of which could in part be inhibited by a regular intake of specific micronutrients.

In 1983 (32) we reported the results of an intervention study employing vitamin C in 51 hypochlorhydric subjects at high risk gastric cancer due either to pernicious anaemia, chronic atrophic gastritis or partial gastrectomy. Fasting gastric juice samples were obtained before, at the end of 4 weeks high dose vitamin C treatment and again 4 weeks after this treatment was discontinued. The following parameters were measured in the gastric juice: pH, NO_2, NOC, total and nitrate-reducing bacterial counts. The mean nitrite and total NOC concentrations were reduced in the group as a whole. The reduction was most marked following partial gastrectomy, even though the gastric pH remained virtually unchanged. Of 220 samples tested in the Ames test system 55 were found to be mutagenic and 42 (72%) of these were obtained when the patients were not taking supplemental vitamin C.

This intervention trial was later extended to include patients with vagotomy for benign peptic ulcer, the data were subsequently re-analysed and presented at the 1989 AGA meeting in Washington (33). At baseline there was a gradient in the median gastric juice NOC levels from the lowest in highly selective vagotomy to the highest in pernicious

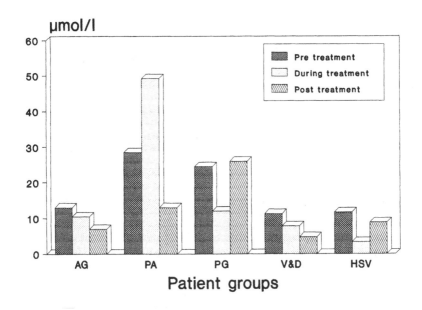

Figure 13: Median NOC levels.

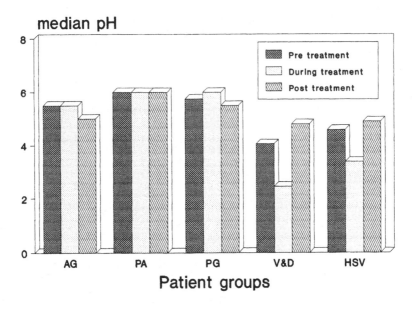

Figure 14: Median intragastric pH.

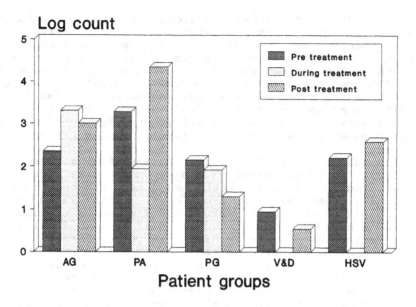

Figure 15: Median NO_2 reducing bacterial log count.

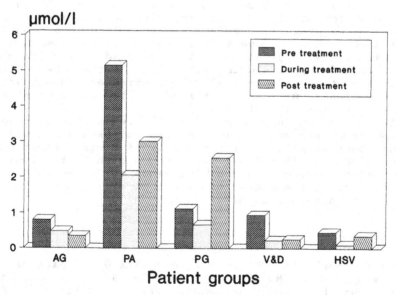

Figure 16: Median NO_2 levels.

anaemia, and with the other surgically treated patients in
between (fig. 13), which correlates absolutely with the
expected change based on progressive hypochlorhydria. An
unexpected fall in the intragastric pH was observed during
the vitamin C treatment period in the vagotomised patients
(fig. 14), resulting in a concurrent inhibition in the
growth of intragastric nitrate reducing microorganisms (fig.
15). All groups showed a fall in the NO_2 concentration
during treatment (fig. 13) and all groups except pernicious
anaemia showed a fall in NOC levels during vitamin C
treatment.

Although the data from these intervention studies are
not conclusive nevertheless they have shown that vitamin C
administration will reduce both endogenous nitrosation and
mutagenicity. Sufficient information is now available about
the probable mechanism of gastric carcinogenesis to suggest
that the intestinal type of GC is well suited for larger
scale intervention studies in high risk GC populations.

The most pertinent observations from this preliminary
analysis of the dietary relations shows a strong protective
role for fresh fruits and salads and in the UK where plasma
vitamin levels were also measured a strong inverse
relationship was observed in the presence of IM and plasma
vitamin C levels consistent with the dietary observations.

Both these sets of observations on the development of IM
and the progression to epithelial dysplasia (ED) suggest
strongly that ascorbic acid should be useful in the
chemoprevention of GC and reinforce already available data.

Since the protective effect of ascorbic acid a powerful
antioxidant, in carcinogenesis is supported by experimental
and human epidemiological data it is planned to institute an
intervention study employing vitamin C as the intervention
agent. The study will be a placebo controlled 2 armed study
and the patients will be stratified by the IM type at the
time of entry into the study.

In conclusion, having outlined the relationship between
diet and pre-cancerous lesions of the stomach and a strong
case has been established for the role of dietary factors in
the aetiology of intestinal type GC and that the logical
further step to reducing the incidence of GC would be the
use of appropriate antioxidants long-term in subjects at
high risk of developing GC.

ACKNOWLEDGMENTS

I wish to thank the CRC for funding the U.K. part of the
ECP/IM study, dr R. Muggli, Hoffman La Roche & Co. for
carrying out the vitamin analyses, Drs CL Walters & PLR
Smith for the N-nitroso compounds and nitrate analyses and
Mrs Belinda Johnston for all the coordinating work in

preparing this paper.

REFERENCES

1. Muir, C., Waterhouse, J., Mack, T., Powell, J. and Whelan, S. (eds) (1987) Cancer Incidence in Five Continents, Vol. V, IARC Sci. Publ. No 75, IARC, LYON.
2. Hill, M. J. (1987) Gastric carcinogenesis: Luminal factors. In Reed, P.I. and Hill, M.J. (eds) Gastric Carcinogenesis, pp. 187-200 (Amsterdam, Excerpta Medica).
3. Lauren, P. (1965) The two histological main types of gastric carcinoma: diffuse and so-called intestinal type. Acta Path. Microbiol Scand, 64, 31-49.
4. Correa, P., Haenszel, W., Cuello, C., Tannenbaum, S. and Archer, M. (1975) A model for gastric cancer epidemiology. Lancet, ii, 58-60.
5. Watt, P. C. H., Straw, J. M., Donaldson, J.D., Patterson, C.C. and Kennedy, T.L. (1984) Relationship between histology and gastric juice pH and nitrite in the stomach after operation for duodenal ulcer. Gut, 25, 246-252.
6. Forman, D., Al-Dabbagh, S. and Doll, R. (1985) Nitrates, nitrites and gastric cancer in Great Britain. Nature, 313, 620-625.
7. Beresford, S. A. (1985) Is nitrate in the drinking water associated with the risk of cancer in the urban UK? Int J Epidemiol, 14, 57-63.
8. Mirvish, S.S. (1985) Gastric cancer and salivary nitrate and nitrite. Nature, 315, 415-462.
9. Tannenbaum, S.R. and Correa, P. (1985) Nitrate and gastric cancer risks. Nature, 317, 675-676.
10. Hill, M.J. (1990) Personal communication.
11. Bogovski, P. and Bogovski, S. (1981) Animal species in which N-nitroso compounds induce cancer. Special report. Int. J. Cancer, 27, 471-474.
12. Schmahl, D. and Scherf, H. R. (1984) Carcinogenic activity of N-nitroso-diethylamine in snakes (Python reticulatus Biodae). In Bartsch, H. , O'Neill, I.K., Von Borstel, R., Miller, C.T. et al. (eds) N-nitroso-compounds: Occurrence, Biological effects and Relevance to Human Cancer, IARC Scient. Publ. 57 pp. 677-682, Lyon, IARC.
13. Winn, D.M. (1984) In Bartsch, H., O'Neill, I.K., Von Borstel, R., Miller, C.T. et al. (eds) N-nitroso-compounds: Occurrence, Biological effects and Relevance to Human Cancer, IARC Scient. Publ. 57 pp. 837-849 (Lyon, IARC).
14. Hicks, R.M., Walters, C.L., Esebai, I., El Aasser, A.-A., El Mersatani, M. and Gough, T.A. (1977)

Demonstration of nitrosamines in human urine. Preliminary observations on a possible aetiology for bladder cancer in association with chronic urinary tract infections. Proc. R. Soc. Med. 70, 413.

15. Young, C.S. (1982) Nitrosamines and other aetiological factors in oesophageal cancer in Northern China. In Magee, R.N (ed.) Banbury Report 12, Nitrosamines and Human Cancer. pp. 487-499 (New York: Cold Spring Harbor Laboratory).

16. Correa, P. (1988) A human model of gastric carcinogenesis. Cancer Res. 48, 3554-3560.

17. Weisburger, J. H. and Horn, C. L. (1982) On the factors associated with oesophageal and gastric cancer in man. In Magee, P.N. (ed.) Banbury Report 12: Nitrosamines and Human Cancer. pp. 523-528 (New York, Cold Spring Harbor Laboratory).

18. Hirayama, T. (1988) Actions suggested by gastric cancer epidemiological studies in Japan. In Reed, P.I. and Hill, M.J. (eds) Gastric Carcinogenesis, pp. 209-227 (Amsterdam: Excerpta Medica).

19. Preussmann, R. and Tricker, A.R. (1988) Endogenous nitrosamine formation and nitrate burden in relation to gastric cancer epidemiology. In Reed, P.I. and Hill, M.J. (eds) Gastric Carcinogenesis, pp. 147-162, (Amsterdam :Excerpta Medica)

20. Block, G. (1989) Vitamin C and cancer : The epidemiological evidence. Proc. International Conference on antioxidant vitamins and beta-carotene in disease prevention. London, October 1989.

21. Ziegler, R.G. (1989) Carotenoid intake and risk of cancer. Proc. International Conference on antioxidant vitamins and beta-carotene in disease prevention. London, October 1989.

22. Stahelin, H. B. (1989) Beta-carotene and cancer prevention: The Basle study. Proc. International Conference on antioxidant vitamins and beta-carotene in disease prevention. London, October 1989.

23. Adam, B., Schlag, P., Friede, P., Preussmann, R. and Eisebrand, G. (1989) Proline is not useful as a chemical probe to measure nitrosation in the gastrointestinal tract of patients with gastric disorders characterised by anacidic conditions. Gut, 30, 1068-1075.

24. Reed, P. I., Haines, K., Smith, P. L. R., Walters, C. L. and House, F.R. (1981) The gastric juice N-nitrosamines in health and gastro-duodenal disease. Lancet, ii, 550-552.

25. Stockbrugger, R. W., Cotton, P. B., Eugenides, N., Bartholomew, B.A., Hill, M.J. and Walters, C.L. (1982) Intragastric nitrites, nitrosamines, and bacterial overgrowth during cimetidine treatment. Gut, 23, 1048-1052.

26. Mirvish, S.S. (1975) Formation of N-nitroso compounds: Chemistry, kinetics and in vivo occurrence. Toxicol Appl Pharmacol, 31, 325-351.

27. Ohshima, H. and Bartsch, H. (1981) Quantitative estimation of endogenous nitrosation in humans by monitoring N-nitrosoproline excreted in the urine. Cancer Res, 41, 3658-3662.

28. West, C. E. and Van Staveren, W. A. (1987) ECP-EURONUT intestinal metaplasia study: Design of the study with special reference to the development and validation of the questionnaire. In Reed, P.I. and Hill, M.J. (eds) Gastric Carcinogenesis, pp. 229-234. (Amsterdam: Excerpta Medica).

29. Judd, P.A. for the ECP-EURONUT intestinal metaplasia study: Design of the study with special reference to the development and validation of the questionnaire. In Reed, P.I. and Hill, M.J. (eds) Gastric Carcinogenesis, (Amsterdam: Excerpta Medica).

30. Hill, M.J. for the ECP-EURONUT intestinal metaplasia study: Design of the study with special reference to the development and validation of the questionnaire. In Reed, P.I. and Hill, M.J. (eds) Gastric Carcinogenesis, (Amsterdam: Excerpta Medica).

31. Kyrtopoulos, S. (1984) Nitrosamines in the environment. Health dangers and intervention possibilities. In Environmental Carcinogens. The problem in Greece. Proc Panhellenic Congress of Greek Society of Preventive Medicine, March 1984.

32. Reed, P. I., Summers, K., Smith, P. L.R., Walters, C.L., Bartholomew, B., Hill, M.J., Vennitt, S., Hornig, D. and Bonjour, J-P. (1983) Effect of ascorbic acid treatment on gastric juice nitrite and N-nitroso compound concentration in achlorhydric subjects. Gut, 24, A492-A493.

33. Reed, P.I., Johnston, B.J., Walters, C.L. and Hill, M.J. (1989) Effect of ascorbic acid on the intragastric environment in patients at increased risk of developing gastric cancer. Gastroenterology, 96, A411.

7

REPRODUCTIVE FACTORS, ORAL CONTRACEPTIVES AND BREAST CANCER: THE IMPORTANCE OF UNIFYING HYPOTHESES

Carlo La Vecchia

Istituto di Recerche Farmacologiche "Mario Negri", 20157 Milano, Italy and Institute of Social and Preventive Medicine, University of Lausanne, 1005 Lausanne, Switzerland

ACKNOWLEDGEMENTS

This work was conducted within the framework of the National Research Council (CNR), Applied Projects "Oncology" (Contract No. 87.01544.44) and "Risk Factors for Disease", and with the contribution of the Italian Association for Cancer Research and the Italian League Against Tumours, Milan. The author wish to thank Ms. A. Rattaz for editorial assistance.

REPRODUCTIVE FACTORS

The relation between breast cancer and hormonal and reproductive factors has been studied extensively, but the evidence is still controversial.

The role of parity and age at first birth has been a topic of debate over the last two decades, since in some studies the risk seemed to be related only to age at first birth and not to parity, in others the only latter variable seemed to influence the risk of breast cancer, while other studies found an independent effect of both variables.

A formal overview of published material (1) indicates that both variables are likely to have an effect on breast cancer risk, but these effects are relatively small and can easily be missed in studies of even several hundred cases.

Overall, among 26 studies considered (2), one found no significant association with parity nor with age at first birth, seven reported an association between age at first birth but not parity, six an inverse relation with parity but not age at first birth, and 12 found both variables independently related with breast cancer risk (Tables 1-3).

Various reasons for these apparent discrepancies could

TABLE 1. Studies showing association between age at first birth but not parity and breast cancer risk.

study, country	Parity					Age at first birth				
	1	2	3	4	>5	<20	20-24	25-29	30-34	>35
MacMahon et al. (12) 7 countries	1*	1.1	1.0	1.0	0.9	1*	1.2	1.6	1.9	2.5
Herity et al. (13) Ireland		1*			0.9	1*		0.9	1.2	2.3
MacMahon et al. (14) Estonia	1*	0.7	0.6	1.3		1*	1.8	2.4	2.4	2.4
Trapido (15) USA	1*		1.0		0.9	1*	1.5	2.1	2.7	
Brinton et al. (16) USA	1*	1.0	1.0	0.9	0.8	1*	1.3	1.7	2.5	
Talamini et al. (17) Italy	1*			0.8		1*		1.3	1.6	
Brignone et al. (18) Italy	1*		1.2		1.1	1*	1.1	1.8	1.9	

* Reference category

70

TABLE 2. Studies showing no significant association between age at first birth and breast cancer risk.

Study, country	Parity					Age at first birth				
	1	2	3	4	>5	<20	20-24	25-29	30-34	>35
Choi et al. (19) Canada	no significant difference					1*	1.0	0.7	0.8	
Adami et al. (20) Sweden	1*	0.7	1.0	0.3	0.4	1*	1.6	2.0	1.0	1.6
Thein et al. (21) Burma	1*			0.6	>6 0.3	1*	0.9	1.0	1.1	1.5
Adami et al. (22) Sweden	1*	0.9	0.6	0.7	0.6	1*	1.0	1.0	1.2	1.7
Paul et al. (23) New Zealand	1*				0.6	1*	1.0	1.0	1.2	
Rosero-Bixby et al.(24) Costa Rica		1*			0.4	1*	1.5		0.8	
Ewertz et al. (25) Denmark	1*	0.9	0.9		0.6	1*	0.9	0.9	1.0	

* Reference category

71

TABLE 3. Studies showing associations between both multiparity and age at first birth and breast cancer risk.

Study, country	Parity					Age at first birth				
	1	2	3	4	>5	<20	20-24	25-29	30-34	>35
Soini (26) Finland	1*	0.9	0.6	0.6	0.4	1*		1.3	1.8	2.0
Tulinius (27) Iceland		1*	0.6		0.5	1*	1.6	2.6	2.5	4.1
Paffenbarger (28) USA	1*	1.0	0.9	0.7		1*	1.6	2.0	2.0	
Bain (29) USA	1*	0.8		0.9	>6 0.7	<20 1*	1.3	1.7	1.9	2.3
Helmrich (30) USA		1*	0.9		0.7	1*	1.2	1.8	1.9	
Toti (31) Italy	1*	1.0	0.8		0.6	1*	1.5	1.6	2.8	
Pathak (32) USA	1*	0.9	0.8	0.7		Directly associated, estimates not given				
Kvale (33,34) Norway	1*	0.9	0.8	0.7	0.5	1*	1.2	1.3	1.4	1.4
La Vecchia (35) Italy		1*		1.1	0.5	1*	1.8	2.2	2.5	
Schatzkin (36) USA		1*		0.9	0.6	1*	1.2	2.0	1.7	
Yuan (37) China	1*	0.7	0.7	0.6	0.4	1*	1.1	1.7	2.7	
Tao (38) China	1	1.1	0.7	0.6	0.6 0.6	1	1.2	1.6	1.4	1.4

* Reference category

be considered, including publication bias, heterogeneity between population, differences between studies in terms of criteria for selection of cases and controls, influence of age and other covariates among which age at diagnosis and the interval between pregnancies and hence the age at subsequent pregnancies may well be of particular importance (3).

Further, the role of chance cannot be dismissed, since the risk estimates of both variables were relatively moderate, the distribution in various strata largely uneven, and the absolute numbers of subjects relatively small in several studies. There is, therefore, ample scope for more formal pooling exercices on the issue, based on the original datasets, in order to derive independently adjusted overall estimates of the separate effects of age at first birth and parity on breast cancer risk, and their interaction.

At present, the conclusions that can be derived from the data considered appear to suggest, from an aetiological viewpoint, that both factors have some independent effect on breast carcinogenesis. From a public health viewpoint, however, age at first birth seems more important, since the trend of increasing risk with older age at first full-term pregnancy is evident and rather linear across all the subsequent levels, while the protection of parity, even in the studies where the association was evident, seems to be quantitatively relevant only for women with four or five births or more.

THE MODIFYING EFFECT OF AGE

It is now clear that age at diagnosis and other time factors have an important modifying effect on the association between reproductive factors and breast cancer. While the protection exerted by age at first birth is observed in various subsequent age groups, parity is associated with elevated breast cancer risk in young women only (i.e, below age 40), with a subsequent cross-over towards a long-term protection in middle age and older women.

Table 4 is derived from a meta analysis of two large case-control studies from Italy, including a total of 4,072 cases and 4,099 controls (4). The effect of age at first birth was consistent among subsequent strata of age, whereas that of parity showed clear interaction with age; multiparous women, in fact, were at elevated risk of breast cancer below age 35, but at reduced risk above age 40. This confirms previous evidence based on vital statistics, case-control and prospective studies of a "crossover" effect of breast cancer incidence around age 40.

Indeed, a further analysis of the same dataset (5) has shown that a full-term pregnancy is followed by a transient

TABLE 4. Relative risks of breast cancer according to parity and age at first birth in separate age strata, Italy, 1972-1986 (Derived from Negri et al. (4)).

Variable	< 35	35-39	Age group (years)			
			40-49	50-59	60-69	>70
Parity						
0*	1	1	1	1	1	1
1	1.6	0.9	0.9	0.8	1.0	0.9
2	1.1	0.6	0.9	0.8	0.9	0.9
3-4	2.2	1.0	0.8	0.6	0.9	0.7
> 5	1.8	1.0	0.6	0.3	0.5	0.4
X21 (trend)	1.9	0.3	4.4	28.0	11.7	19.6
	(NS)**	(NS)	(p=0.04)	(p<0.001)	(p<0.001)	(p<0.001)
Age (years) at first live birth						
< 22*	1	1	1	1	1	1
22-24	1.2	1.0	1.7	1.1	1.2	1.5
25-27	1.4	1.4	1.8	1.4	1.2	2.1
> 28	2.0	2.2	2.1	2.1	1.5	2.3
Nulliparae	0.8	1.6	2.0	2.0	1.5	2.4
X21(trend)#	4.3	8.4	18.9	39.9	8.8	24.0
	(p=0.04)	(p=0.004)	(p<0.001)	(p<0.001)	(p=0.003)	(p<0.001)

* Reference category
** NS, not significant
# Nulliparae excluded

increase in the risk of breast cancer, which for some time counteracts and overcomes the protective effect of pregnancy : compared with women whose last birth occurred more than 10 years in advance, the relative risk was 2.7 during the three years following a term pregnancy (Table 5).

TABLE 5. Relative risks of breast cancer among 573 cases and 570 controls aged <50 who had two or more children (Derived from Bruzzi et al. (5))

Years since last birth	Relative risk (95% confidence intervals)
> 10	1 (reference)
7 - < 10	1.4 (1.0-1.9)
3 - < 7	1.8 (1.1-2.9)
< 3	2.7 (1.3-5.4)
x^2_1 for trend	9.9 (p < 0.01)

These findings fit the predictions from the standard multistage theory of carcinogenesis (6), as well as from a more formal two stage model of breast carcinogenesis proposed by Moolgavkar et al. (7) to interpret epidemiological features of breast cancer. Within the two stage model, it can be assumed that a pregnancy acts as an anti-initiator, by reducing the pool of susceptible stem cells through differentiation, and as a promoter, by expanding the clone of initiated cells. Different hormonal mechanisms are likely to have a role in these two effects (8). The model predicts a long-term protection inversely proportional to the age at pregnancy and a short-term increase in risk that in relative terms is independent of age at pregnancy. These were exactly the results obtained from direct epidemiological observation and underline the importance of integrating biological and statistical models to interpret epidemiological data.

ORAL CONTRACEPTIVES

Despite the large number of published studies, the debate on the possible association between oral contraceptives and

TABLE 6: Summary tabulation of studies of oral contraceptives and breast cancer.

Author, Reference Country	Type of study Comments	Number of cases (age)	Relative risk for oral contraceptives	
			ever use	longest use
Henderson (39), USA	Case-control based on pathology records. Approx. 70% of breast cancers interviewed. Controls from the same physicians, matched for age.	308 (<65)	0.7	–
Paffenbarger (40) USA	Case-control hospital-based. Controls from medical and surgical services. Cases and controls interviewed at home.	452 (<50)	1.1	1.7
Sartwell (41) USA	Case-control hospital-based. Controls from surgical & medical wards, interviewed in hospital.	284 (20-74)	0.9	1.0
Kelsey (42) USA	Case-control hospital-based. Controls from surgical services matched for age, marital status, race and education.	99 (20-44)	1.6	–
Ravnihar (43) Yugoslavia	Case-control hospital-based. Controls admitted to the same medical center for a wide spectrum of conditions.	190 (20-49)	0.9	–
Jick (44) USA	Historical cohort + case-control. From the Puget Sound Group Health Cooperative. See ref. 69.	132 <46y (<56) 16-55y	0.8 8.0	– –

Study	Description	No. (age)		
Paffenbarger (28) USA	Case-control hospital based. Controls from medical & surgical services. Participation rate about 70%.	378* 1038**	1.1 1.2	1.1 1.5
Kelsey (45) USA	Case-control hospital-based. Controls from surgical services. Participation rate, 74% cases, 72% controls.	332 (45–74)	0.9	0.4
RCPG (46) UK	Cohort. Increased risk in young women (aged 30 to 34, RR=3.3). See ref.66.	133	1.2	–
Vessey (47) UK	Cohort. Report from the Oxford-Family Planning Association (FPA) Study. See ref. 67.	72	1.0	–
Trapido (48) USA	Cohort. Follow-up study from the 1969 Boston residence list. Elevated risk in selected subgroups (e.g., nulliparae).	622 (25–50)	0.8	0.9
Pike (49) USA	Case-control population-based. Cases identified through the Los Angeles County Cancer Registry. Response rate, 56%. One neighbourhood & one friend control per case. Elevated risk for use before first birth.	163 (<32)	1.2	2.2
Harris (50) USA	Case-control population-based. Overall response rate, 64% cases, 92% controls. Elevated risk for use in pre-menopausal women aged $\geq$ 40.	112 (35–54)	1.0	0.8

Study	Description	No. (age range)		
Brinton (51) USA	Case-control from the Breast Cancer. Detection Demonstration Project (BCDDP). Participation rate 86% cases, 74% controls. White women only with no history of artificial menopause. Elevated risk for use after age 40. See ref. 72.	962	1.1	1.0
Lubin (52) Canada	Case-control population-based. Significant association before age 45.	557 (30-80)	0.9 (former users) 1.7 (recent users)	– –
Vessey (53,54) UK	Case-control hospital-based. Married women with breast cancer & acute surgical or medical conditions (controls). Interaction with stage (less advanced for users) but not with other variables considered.	1176 (16-50)	1.0	1.0
Pike (55) USA	Case-control population-based. See Pike et al. (49), but neighbourhood controls only. Elevated risk for use before age 25 or first birth & high progestogen OC.	314 (<37)	–	4.9
Hennekens (56) USA	Case-control from the Nurses Health Study. Prevalent cases from the Nurses Health Study. Elevated risk in the subgroup aged 50-55 at diagnosis (7 observed vs 2 expected).	989 (30-55)	1.0	0.7
Rosenberg (57) USA	Case-control hospital-based. From the Slone Epidemiology Unit dataset. Elevated risk for women aged 30 to 39 (RR=1.3).	1191 (20-59)	0.9	0.8

78

Study	Description	Number (age)		
Talamini (17) Italy	Case-control hospital-based. Controls from orthopaedical, surgical & medical wards. Participation rate 99%. Low prevalence of OC use.	373 (27-79)	0.7	--
The Cancer and Steroid Hormone Study (58) USA	Case-control population-based. From eight areas of the SEER Program. Controls selected through random-digit dialing (participation rate 83%).	4711 (20-54)	1.0	0.6
Miller (59) USA	Case-control hospital-based. Further analysis on the Slone Epidemiology Unit dataset. No evidence of increased risk in any subgroup.	521 (<45)	1.0	1.4
Lipnick (60) USA	Cohort. Incident cases from the Nurses Health Study.	529 (30-55)	1.0	1.3
La Vecchia (61) Italy	Case-control hospital-based. Controls admitted for acute conditions to the same network of hospitals. Participation rate 98%.	776 (<60)	1.1	1.1
Paul (23) New Zealand	Case-control population-based. National study. Elevated risk for long-term use among women aged 35 or less at diagnosis.	433 (25-54)	0.9	1.0
Meirik (62) Sweden, Norway	Case-control population-based. Participation rate 89% cases, 85% controls (Sweden): 92% cases, 71% controls (Norway). Risk related with duration of use, but not age at first OC use or latency from first use.	422 (<49)	--	2.2

Study	Description	Number		
Jick (69) USA	Case-control. Data collected through interview from the Puget Sound Group Health Cooperative. Two studies pooled, one with population & one with hospital controls. No evidence of association for any of the variables considered.	127 (<43)	0.9	1.4
UK National Case-Control Study Group (70) UK	Case-control population-based. Controls from General Practitioners (GP) lists. Data collected by interview & validated through an independent study on GP records. Response rate 72% for cases, 89% for controls. Direct relation with duration but not any other variable.	755 (<36)	1.4	1.7
Olsson (71) Sweden	Case-control population-based. Data collected by a physician during hospital admission for cases, by interviewers for controls.	174*	1.8	1.8
Standford (72) USA	Case-control from the BCDDP. Interaction with history of breast biopsy and stage of the disease.	2022	1.0	0.7
Romieu (73) USA	Cohort. Update of incident cases from the Nurses Health Study. RR=1.5 (95% CI=1.1-1.2) among current users, but no relationship with duration or other time factors considered.	1799 (30-64)	1.1	–
La Vecchia (61) Italy	Case-control hospital-based. Update of La Vecchia et al, 1976. Recall bias suggested as an explanation for the inconsistent duration-risk relationship.	1351 (<60)	1.3	1.0

* pre-menopausal; ** post-menopausal.

breast cancer is far from settled. The overall evidence, so far, is reassuring: ecological comparisons and temporal trends indicate that, to date, there is no consistent evidence that breast cancer rates have been substantially influenced in any group by the widespread use of oral contraceptives in Western countries. Most case-control and cohort studies (see Table 6 for a summary tabulation), as well as a formal overview (9), based on 16 studies and over 12,000 cases, indicate that breast cancer risk is not higher among ever-users of oral contraceptives than in never-users: the summary RR was 1.0, with a very narrow confidence interval (0.9 to 1.1), and no significant heterogeneity between studies.

There is, however, a subgroup of women in whom positive association between oral contraceptives and breast cancer cannot easily be dismissed as due to chance or bias alone. These are younger (i.e. below age 35 or perhaps up to age 45), long-term oral contraceptive users among whom all (16/16) studies included in Table 7 found relative risks above unity.

TABLE 7. Long-term oral contraceptive use and breast cancer risk in young women.

Study, ref.	Age Group	Relative risk estimate for long term use
Lubin et al. (52)	30-40	1.2
Pike et al. (55)	< 37	4.9
Rosenberg et al. (57)	< 40	1.3
Stadel et al. (74)	< 45	1.3
Meirik et al. (62)	< 40	2.1
La Vecchia et al. (61)	< 45	1.2
Paul et al. (23)	< 35	4.6
McPherson et al. (64)	< 45	2.6
Ravnihar et al. (65)	< 45	2.3
Kay & Hannaford (66)	< 35	2.4*
Miller et al. (68)	< 45	4.1
Jick et al. (69)	< 43	1.4
U.K. National Case-control Study Group (70)	< 36	1.8
Olsson et al. (71)	premenopause	1.8
Romieu et al. (73)	premenopause	1.4(current) - 1.1 (past)

* Ever use

81

This has led to two different types of speculations : i) that long-term use of oral contraceptives at early ages induces unfavourable modifications in the breast, or ii) that the impact of these modifications (or, more in general, of the pill on breast carcinogenesis) may become appreciable only after a long "latent period" and hence that we are now observing only the start of a potential future pill-induced breast cancer epidemic.

At present, however, this is essentially a theoretical scenario, with many others being equally plausible. Besides pharmacological and biological considerations, there is direct epidemiological evidence that the effect of oral contraceptives on various female-hormone-related neoplasms is similar to that of pregnancy : in fact, the pill lowers the risk of ovarian and endometrial cancer, and probably increases that of cervical cancer. Along this same line, the elevated breast cancer risk for long-term oral contraceptive users at younger ages, even if confirmed, would not necessarily indicate that the same excess risk will be reproduced at later ages. In fact, various hypotheses seem equally reasonable, including the persistence of these increased risks, their flattening off, or even their reversal in the medium-long term (10).

CURRENT RESEARCH QUESTIONS ON ORAL CONTRACEPTIVES AND BREAST CANCER

The role of various time factors in the relationship between oral contraceptives and breast cancer should be further investigated. These include calendar period of diagnosis, age at diagnosis, age at starting and stopping use, duration of use, time since first and last use, and calendar period of use.

These time factors are clearly interrelated, and it is consequently difficult to disentangle the separate effect of each factor. For instance, when age at diagnosis and duration are defined, age at starting tends to be defined as well, and this is strongly correlated with calendar period of use, and hence type of preparation as well.

For some of these temporal relationships, there is an inevitable paucity or absence of information in the studies conducted to date. For instance, while an association between long-term oral contraceptive use at younger age and breast cancer risk has been observed in women below age 35 or 40, no data are available on the possible impact of such a use on middle age or older women simply because oral contraceptives were not avalaible when those generations of women were in their younger age. Thus, reliable information on the impact of oral contraceptives on women aged 40 to 60 is now of outstanding importance.

Type of preparation is another related question to be investigated, since there is some indication that newer preparations are less consistently associated with breast cancer risk, even at younger age.

The potential role of some covariates may deserve some attention, although there is at present little convincing evidence of association in any particular sub-group. Some of these covariates, such as benign breast disease or family history, may nonetheless be of interest as interaction/modifying factors.

CONCLUSION: THE IMPORTANCE OF UNIFYING HYPOTHESES

In the absence of a precise understanding of the underlying biological mechanism, epidemiology can nonetheless try to develop integrated hypotheses for hormonal and reproductive factors in breast carcinogenesis, which could be tested in the large amount of data already collected. Further, the apparent discrepancies between published data should not only be considered in terms of chance or bias (11), but also viewed within the framework of the complex, and sometimes contradictory, age and time effects of various (hormone-related) risk factors in breast carcinogenesis (10).

The elucidation of the timing of the oral contraceptives-breast cancer relationship is, of course, a crucial point in defining the long-term implications of oral contraceptives in breast cancer risk, and hence ultimately for quantifying any risk-benefit analysis of oral contraceptives and disease. Only future studies, however, will have the possibility of studying the long-term impact of early, long lasting oral contraceptive use, and hence to provide reliable assessment of this issue.

REFERENCES

1. La Vecchia, C., Negri, E., and Boyle, P. (1989). Reproductive factors and breast cancer : an overview. Soz Preventiv med, 34, 101-107.
2. La Vecchia, C., Parazzini, F., Negri, E et al. (1989) Breast cancer and combined oral contraceptives : an Italian case control study. **Eur J Cancer Clin Oncol**, **25**, 1613-1618.
3. Negri, E., La Vecchia, C., Duffy, S.W., Bruzzi, P., Parazzini, F. and Day, N.E. (1990) Age at first and second birth and breast cancer risk in biparous women. Int J Cancer, (in press).
4. Negri, E. , La Vecchia, C., Bruzzi, P., Dardanoni, G., Decarli, A., Palli, D., Parazzini, F. and Rosselli del

Turco, M. (1988). Risk factors for breast cancer: pooled results from three Italian case-control studies. Am J Epidemiol, 128, 1207-1215.

5. Bruzzi, P., Negri, E., La Vecchia, C., Decarli, A., Palli, D., Parazzini, P. and Rosselli del Turco, M. (1988) Short-term increase in risk of breast cancer after full-term pregnancy. Br Med J, 297, 1096-1098.

6. Day, N. E. and Brown, C.C. (1980). Multistage models and primary prevention of cancer. JNCI, 64, 977-989.

7. Moolgavkar, S. H., Day, N. E. and Stevens, R. G. (1980). Two-stage model for carcinogenesis: epidemiology of breast cancer in females. JNCI, 65, 559-569.

8. Russo, I. H. and Russo, J. (1986). From pathogenesis to hormone prevention of mammary carcinogenesis. Cancer Surv, 5, 649-670.

9. Prentice, R. L., Thomas, D.B. (1987). On the epidemiology of oral contraceptives and disease. Adv Cancer Res, 49, 285-401.

10. La Vecchia, C., Bruzzi, P. and Boyle, P. (1990). Some further consideration on the role of oral contraceptives in breast carcinogenesis. Tumori, (in press).

11. Skegg, D.C.G. (1988). Reviews and Commentary. Potential for bias in case-control studies of oral contraceptives and breast cancer. Am J Epidemiol, 127, 205-212.

12. MacMahon, B., Cole, P., Lin, M., Lowe, C.R., Mirra, A.P., Ravnihar, B. Salber, E.J., et al. (1970). Age at first birth and breast cancer risk. Bull WHO, 43, 209-221.

13. Herity, B. A., O'Halloran, M.J., Bourke, G.J., Wilson--Davis, K. (1975). A study of breast cancer in Irish women. Brit J Prev Soc Med, 29, 178-181.

14. MacMahon, B., Purde, M., Cramer, D. and Hint, E. (1982). Association of breast cancer risk with age at first and subsequent births: a study in the population of the Estonian Republic. JNCI, 69, 1035-1038.

15. Trapido, E.J. (1983). Age at first birth, parity and breast cancer risk. Cancer, 51, 946-948.

16. Brinton, L.A., Hoover, R. and Fraumeni, J.F. Jr. (1983). Reproductive factors in the aetiology of breast cancer. Br J Cancer, 47, 757-762.

17. Talamini, R., La Vecchia, C., Franceschi, S. et al. (1985) Reproductive and hormonal factors and breast cancer in a Northern Italian population. Int J Epidemiol, 14, 70-74.

18. Brignone, G., Cusimano, R., Dardanoni, G., Gugliuzza, M., Lanzarone, F., Scibilia, V. and Dardanoni, L. (1987). A case-control study on breast cancer risk factors in a Southern European population. Int J Epidemiol, 16, 356-361.

19. Choi, N. W., Howe, G. R., Miller, A.B. et al. (1978). An epidemiologic study of breast cancer. Am J Epidemiol,

107, 510-521.

20. Adami, H. O., Rimsten, A., Stenkvist, B. and Vegelius, J. (1978). Reproductive history and risk of breast cancer. Cancer, 41, 747-757.

21. Thein-Hlaing, Thein-Maung-Myint. (1978). Risk factors of breast cancer in Burma. Int J Cancer, 21, 432-437.

22. Adami, H.O., Hansen, J., Jung, B. and Rimsten, A.J. (1980). Age at first birth, parity and risk of breast cancer in a Swedish population. Br J Cancer, 42, 651-658.

23. Paul, C., Skegg, D.C.G, Spears, G.F.S. and Kaldor, J.M. (1986). Oral contraceptives and breast cancer: a national study. Br Med J; 293, 723-726.

24. Rosero-Bixby, L., Oberle, M. W. and Lee, N.C. (1987). Reproductive history and breast cancer in a population of high fertility, Costa Rica, 1984-85. Int J Cancer, 40, 747-754.

25. Ewertz, M. and Duffy, S.W. (1988). Risk of breast cancer in relation to reproductive factors in Denmark. Br J Cancer, 58, 99-104.

26. Soini, I. (1977). Risk factors of breast cancer in Finland. Int J Epidemiol, 6, 365-373.

27. Tulinius, H., Day, N. E., Johannesson, G., Bjarnason, O. and Gozales, M. (1978). Reproductive factors and risk of breast cancer in Iceland. Int J Cancer, 21, 724-730.

28. Paffenbarger, R. S. Jr, Kampert, J.B. and Chang, H.G. (1980). Characteristics that predict risk of breast cancer before and after the menopause. Am J Epidemiol, 112, 258-268.

29. Bain, Ch., Willett, W., Rosner, B., Speizer, F.E., Belanger, Ch., and Hennekens, C.H. (1981). Early age at first birth and decreased risk of breast cancer. Am J Epidemiol, 114, 705-709.

30. Helmrich, S. P., Shapiro, S., Rosenberg, L., Kaufman, D.W., Slone, D., Bain, Ch., Miettinen, O. et al. (1983). Risk factors for breast cancer. Am J Epidemiol, 117, 35-45.

31. Toti, A., Agugiaro, S., Amadori, D. et al. (1986). Breast cancer risk factors in Italian women: a multicentric case-control study. Tumori, 72, 241-249.

32. Pathak, D. R., Speizer, F.E., Willet, W.C., Rosner, B. and Lipnick, R.J. (1986). Parity and breast cancer risk: possible effect on age at diagnosis. Int J Cancer, 37, 21-25.

33. Kvale, G. and Heuch, I. (1987 a). A prospective study of reproductive factors and breast cancer. II. Age at first and last birth. Am J Epidemiol, 126, 842-850.

34. Kvale, G., Heuch, I. and Eide, G.E. (1987 b). A prospective study of reproductive factors and breast cancer. I. Parity. Am J Epidemiol, 126, 831-841.

35. La Vecchia, C., Decarli, A., Parazzini, F., Gentile, A., Negri, E., Cecchetti, G. and Franceschi, S. (1987).

General epidemiology of breast cancer in Northern Italy. Int J Epidemiol, 16, 347-355.

36. Schatzkin, A., Palmer, J. E., Rosenberg, L. et al. (1987). Risk factors for breast cancer in black women. JNCI, 78, 213-217.

37. Yuan, J. M., Yu, M.C., Ross, R.K., Gao, Y.T. and Henderson, B.E. (1988). Risk factors for breast cancer in Chinese women in Sanghai. Cancer Res, 48, 1949-1953.

38. Tao, S.C., Yu, M.C., Ross, R.K. and Xiu, K.W. (1988). Risk factors for breast cancer in Chinese women of Beijing. Int J Cancer, 42, 495-498.

39. Henderson, B. E., Powell, D., Rosario, I. et al. (1974). An epidemiologic study of breast cancer. J Natl Cancer Inst, 53, 609-614.

40. Paffenbarger, R.S. Jr, Fasal, E., Simmons, M.E. and Kampert, J.B. (1977). Cancer risk as related to use of oral contraceptives during fertile years. Cancer, 39, 1887-1891.

41. Sartwell, P.E., Arthes, F.G. and Tonascia, J.A. (1977). Exogenous hormones, reproductive history and breast cancer. J Natl Cancer Inst, 59, 1589-1592.

42. Kelsey, J. L., Holford, T. R., White, C., Mayer, E. S., Kilty, S.E. and Acheson, R.M. (1978). Oral contraceptives and breast cancer. Am J Epidemiol, 107, 236-244.

43. Ravnihar, B., Seigel, D.G. and Lindtner, J. (1979). An epidemiologic study of breast cancer and benign breast neoplasias in relation to the oral contraceptive and estrogen use. Europ J Cancer, 15, 395-405.

44. Jick, H., Walker, A.M., Watkins, R.N. et al. (1980). Oral contraceptives and breast cancer. Am J Epidemiol, 112, 577-585.

45. Kelsey, J.L., Fischer, D. B., Holford, T.R. et al. (1981). Exogenous estrogens and other factors in the epidemiology of breast cancer. JNCI, 67, 327-333.

46. Royal College of General Practitioners. (1981). Breast cancer and oral contraceptives: findings in Royal College of General Practitioners'study. Br Med J, 282, 2089-2093.

47. Vessey, M. P., McPherson, K. and Doll, R. (1981). Breast cancer and oral contraceptives: findings in Oxford-Family Planning Association contraceptive study. Br J Med, 282, 2093-2094.

48. Trapido, E.J. (1981). A Prospective cohort study of oral contraceptives and breast cancer. JNCI, 67, 1011-1015.

49. Pike, M. C., Henderson, B.E., Casagrande, J.T., Rosario, I. and Gray, G.E. (1981). Oral contraceptive use and early abortion as risk factors for breast cancer in young women. Br J Cancer, 43, 72-76.

50. Harris, N. V., Weiss, N. S., Francis, A.M. and Polissar, L. (1982). Breast cancer in relation to patterns of oral

contraceptive use. Am J Epidemiol, 116, 643-651.

51. Brinton, L. A., Hoover, R., Szklo, M. and Fraumeni, J.F Jr. (1982). Oral contraceptives and breast cancer. Int J Epidemiol, 11, 316-322.

52. Lubin, J.H., Burns, P.E., Blot, W.J. et al. (1982). Risk factors for breast cancer in women in Northern Alberta, Canada, as related to age at diagnosis. JNCI, 68, 211-217.

53. Vessey, M. P., McPherson, K., Yeates, D. and Doll, R. (1982). Oral contraceptive use and abortion before first term pregnancy in relation to breast cancer risk. Br J Cancer, 45, 327-331.

54. Vessey, M. Baron, J., Doll, R., McPherson, K. and Yeates, D. (1983). Oral contraceptives and breast cancer: final report of an epidemiological study. Br J Cancer, 47, 455-462.

55. Pike, M. C., Henderson, B.E., Krailo, M.D., Duke, A. and Roy, S. (1983) Breast cancer in young women and use of oral contraceptives: possible modifying effect of formulation and age at use. Lancet, ii, 926-930.

56. Hennekens, C. H., Speizer, F. E., Lipnick, R. J. et al. (1984). A case-control study of oral contraceptive use and breast cancer. JNIC, 72, 39-42.

57. Rosenberg, L., Miller, D.R., Kaufman, D. W. et al. (1984) Breast cancer and oral contraceptive use. Am J Epidemiol, 119, 167-176.

58. The Cancer and Steroid Hormone Study of the Centers for Disease Control and the National Institute of Child Health and Human Development. (1986). Oral-contraceptive use and the risk of breast cancer. N Engl J Med, 315, 405-411.

59. Miller, D.R., Rosenberg, L., Kaufman, D.W., Schottenfeld, D., Stolley, P.D. and Shapiro, S. (1986). Breast cancer risk in relation to early oral contraceptive use. Obstet Gynecol, 68, 863.

60. Lipnick, R.J., Buring, J.E., Hennekens, C.H. et al. (1986). Oral contraceptives and breast cancer. A prospective cohort study. JAMA, 255, 58-61.

61. La Vecchia, C., Decarli, A., Fasoli, M. et al. (1986). Oral contraceptives and cancers of the breast and of the female genital tract. Interim results from a case-control study. Br J Cancer, 54, 311-317.

62. Meirik, O., Lund, E., Adami, H. O., Bergstrom, R., Christoffersen, T. and Bergsjo, P. (1986). Oral contraceptive use and breast cancer in young women. Lancet, ii, 650-654.

63. Lee, N. C., Rosero-Bixby, L., Oberle, M. W., Grimaldo, C., Whatley, A.S. and Rovira; E.Z. (1987). A case-control study of breast cancer and hormonal contraception in Costa Rica. JNCI, 79, 1247-1254.

64. McPherson, K. M., Vessey, M.P., Neil, A., Doll, R.,

Jones, L. and Roberts, M. (1987). Early oral contraceptive use and breast cancer : results of another case-control study. Br J Cancer, 56, 653-660.

65. Ravnihar, B., Primic Zakelj, M., Kosmeli, K. and Stare, J. (1988). A case-control study of breast cancer in relation to oral contraceptive use in Slovenia. Neoplasma, 35, 109-121.

66. Kay, C. R. and Hannaford, P.C. (1988). Breast cancer and the pill - a further report from the Royal College of General Practitioners' oral contraception study. Br J Cancer, 58, 675-680.

67. Vessey, M.P., McPherson, K., Villard-Mackintosh, L., and Yeates, D. (1989). Oral contraceptives and breast cancer: latest findings in a large cohort study. Br J Cancer, 59, 613-617.

68. Miller, D. R., Rosenberg, L., Kaufman, D. W., Stolley, P., Warshauer, M.E. and Shapiro, S. (1989). Breast cancer before age 45 and oral contraceptive use: new findings. Am J Epidemiol, 129, 269-280.

69. Jick, S. S., Walker, A. M., Stergachis, A. and Jick, H. (1989). Oral contraceptives and breast cancer. Br J Cancer, 59, 618-621.

70. UK National case-Control Study Group. (1989). Oral contraceptive use and breast cancer risk in young women. Lancet, i, 974-982.

71. Olsson, H., Moller, T.R. and Ranstam, J. (1989). Early oral contraceptive use and breast cancer among premenopausal women: final report from a study in Southern Sweden. JNCI, 81, 1000-1004.

72. Standford, J. L., Brinton, L.A. and Hoover, R.N. (1989). Oral contraceptives and breast cancer: results from an expanded case-control study. Br J Cancer, 60, 375-381.

73. Romieu, I., Willett, W. C., Colditz, G. A. et al. (1989). Prospective study of oral contraceptive use and risk of breast cancer in women. JNCI, 81, 1313-1321.

74. Stadel, B. V., Rubin, G. L., Webster, L. A. et al. (1985). Oral contraceptives and breast cancer in young women. Lancet, ii, 970-973.

8

FEMALE HORMONES: FOR WHICH CANCERS DO THEY MATTER ?

Silvia Franceschi
Epidemiology Unit, Aviano Cancer Center, Italy.
Chairman of the Hormones and Sexual Factors and Cancer ECP Working Group,
European Organisation for Cooperation in Cancer Prevention Studies, Brussels,
Belgium

INTRODUCTION

Changes in a woman's body resulting from menstrual cycles,
pregnancy, childbirth, lactation and use of exogenous female
hormones are not commonly considered "environmental"
factors. They are, however, environmental in origin, in so
far as they are not solely the product of the individual's
own genetic material, and they were certainly regarded as
"extrinsic factors" by the World Health Organisation (1),
expert committee on the prevention of cancer, which defined
extrinsic factors as including "modifying factors" that
favour neoplasia of apparently intrinsic origin (e.g.
hormone unbalances). Accordingly, Doll & Peto (2) include
them among theoritically avoidable causes of cancer, also on
the basis of the wide variations of presumably
hormone-dependent tumours from community to community. Doll
& Peto (2), only considering cancers of the breast,
endometrium and ovary (i.e. 29% of United States (US) female
cancer deaths and 13% of all US cancer deaths) estimated as
approximately 7% the proportion of cancer deaths avoidable
by control of the causes linked to endogenous hormones (i.e.
menstrual and reproductive factors) and exogenous ones,
chiefly oral contraceptives (OCs). Due, however, to
limitations in presently available knowledge on mechanisms
of hormonal carcinogenesis, not to speak of feasible
preventive approaches, such a percentage was considered very
imprecise. Furthermore, as Doll & Peto (2) emphasize,
hormonal factors may well interact with dietary habits in a
way that is still largely obscure (e.g. the diet may affect
cancer risk by a hormonal mechanism while female hormones
have clear implications in the metabolism and availability
of several nutrients). It is thus difficult to estimate the
extent of overlap between the percentage of cancer
preventable by dietary modification and that attributable to

hormonal mechanisms.

It is, furthermore, worth remembering that an interesting property of hormone-dependent tumours is that, in sharp contrast with most common epithelial malignancies, they all show a clear decrease in the rate of increase around the menopause, as if ceasing menstrual activity reduced risk (3,4).

The present paper will attempt to establish for which neoplasms the aetiologic role of female hormones can be considered established. It will not include breast cancer epidemiology, described elsewhere in the present volume, nor will it try to give a comprehensive review of all available epidemiological knowledge. It will instead focus on those aspects which provide the most interesting clues for future research and prevention. For this reason, a large part of it will deal with OCs, the potential adverse effects of which have received unprecedent attention both by the medical profession and the general public (5).

OVARIAN CANCER

Number of pregnancies

Nulliparity and, even earlier, single marital status (6) have been very consistently related to high risk of ovarian cancer. A strong inverse association between completed family size and mortality from ovarian cancer in different countries and for successive cohorts in the same country has been reported (7). The most debated issue is whether nulliparity and low parity per se or difficulty in conceiving facilitates the development of ovarian cancer. Unfortunately, infertility cannot be measured accurately in most epidemiological studies (8). Many infertile women do not seek medical care for this problem; even more women receive only an incomplete and inconclusive evaluation of the causes of their infertility and/or are unable to report accurately on them.

Some studies suggest, however, that pregnancies exert per se a favourable influence in risk of ovarian cancer. Of twenty studies that have examined the question (6,9-26) showed a further decline in risk associated with full-term pregnancies beyond the first one, thus suggesting that additional risk reduction was conferred by events accompanying each pregnancy. Table 1 summarizes the relative risk estimates from all studies allowing an assessment of the effect of number of pregnancies and at first pregnancy in parous women only (6,9,11-13,16-22,24-26). Investigations which included, as control group, other hormone-dependent female tumours were not considered.

90

TABLE 1: Studies on ovarian cancer reporting relative risk estimates for both parity and age at first birth.

Author	Parity					Age at first birth (yrs)				
	1	2	3	4	5	<20	20-24	25-29	30-34	≥35
Wynder (6)	1	0.8	0.8	1.2	0.8					
Joly (9)	2.1		1.3	1		1	1.4		2.3	
Casagrande (11)	1		0.8							
McGowan (12)	1		1.6	0.3		1	0.7		1.4	
Hildreth (13)	1	0.6	1.0	0.5		1	1.9	3.0	2.5	
Cramer a (16)	1		0.5	0.5		1		1.1	1.2	
b	1		0.5	0.5		1		1.0	1.0	
Risch (17)	1		0.8							
La Vecchia a (18)	1.9		1.7	1		1	2.7	3.2	4.0	
b	1.3		1.2	1		1	2.5	2.8	3.3	
Nasca (19)	1	1.0	1.0	0.8		1	0.7	0.6	0.6	1.1
Tzonou (20)		1		0.7						
Lesher a (21)	1	0.9	0.7	0.6		1	0.8	1.2	1.2	
b	1	0.9	0.7	0.5		1	0.8	1.1	0.9	
Voigt a (22)	1	0.9	0.7	0.8		1	1.0	0.8	1.2	
b	1	0.8	0.7	0.6		1	0.9	0.6	1.0	
Mori (24)	1		1.1	0.4						
Kvale** a (25)	1.5	1.0	0.9	0.8	0.6	0.7	0.9	0.9	1.4	1.0
b	1.4	1.0	0.9	0.9	0.7	0.8	1.0	0.9	1.3	0.8
Wu (26)	1	0.9	0.9			1	1.3	1.0	1.3	

* Reference category; p < 0.05; (a) Unadjusted; (b) Adjusted for parity or age at first birth, as appropriate; ** Cohort study

It is clear that reduction in risk deriving from pregnancies beyond the first one is very weak. Partly on account of limited study sizes, it reached statistical significance in only three investigations (13,16,25).

Results on the influence of incomplete pregnancies, either terminated with a voluntary or spontaneous abortion, are inconclusive. Some authors (25), however, reported that the risk of ovarian cancer was also weakly lowered among women having experienced an abortion.

Age at first pregnancy

The suggestion that early age at first pregnancy may also protect against ovarian cancer came from four case-control studies (9,12,13,18). Since multiply pregnant women usually start reproduction early in their life, independent effects of age at first pregnancy and number of pregnancies are difficult to establish. La Vecchia et al. (18) found a significant excess risk associated with late age at first birth after adjustment for parity. Conversely, low parity was not significantly associated with ovarian cancer risk after adjustment for age at first birth (18). In three case-control studies (16,21,22) and one prospective investigation (25) no relationship with age at first birth remained after adjustment for parity. Several other investigations did not find a consistent increase in risk of ovarian cancer with increasing age at first pregnancy (16,19). The possibility of such an association is further weakened by the aforementioned correlation study (7) where no association with age at first birth or average age at childbirth could be seen.

In conclusion, the effect of age at first pregnancy on ovarian cancer risk, if any, must be weak. However, it is worth remembering that the relative risk estimates for increasing number of children, after exclusion of nulliparous women, also tend to be very close to unity and in most instances are not significantly below it. This issue, therefore, in addition to that concerning the separate effect of parity and fertility, deserves larger and better designed studies, particularly for its potential in elucidating the mechanisms of ovarian carcinogenesis.

Oral contraceptives and ovarian cancer

Epidemiological evidence on OCs and ovarian cancer is very convincing. Thirteen out of 14 studies (10,11,13,15,20-,27-35) (Table 2) found relative risks below unity, the sole apparent outlier being a study conducted in China (33) and including only 21 pill users among the cases and 12 among the controls. The overall estimate of protection was of approximately 40%, and a strong inverse relationship with duration of use. The protection has been shown to persist for some time (at least ten years) after pills use has ceased.

From a biological viewpoint, the beneficial effect of OCs on ovarian cancer risk has been interpreted chiefly in the framework of the "incessant ovulation theory" (11,36). Ovario-stasis, induced by OCs as well as by pregnancy and menopause, avoids the exposure of ovarian epithelium to recurrent trauma and contact with follicular fluid.

Since the incidence of ovarian, as opposed, for instance, to endometrial cancer, is already appreciable in middle age, and survival is substantially lower, the protection attributable to OC use corresponds to a number of deaths that is far from negligible (i.e. probably several hundreds per year in countries like Britain, where OC use has been frequent for a long time).

TABLE 2: Relative risk of ovarian carcinoma in relation to oral contraceptive (OC) use in different studies.

Study	Relative risk (RR) in ever vs never OC users (95% confidence interval)
Newhouse (10)	0.6 (0.3-1.1)
Casagrande (11)	0.7 (0.4-1.1)
Willet (28)	0.8 (0.4-1.5)
Hildreth (13)	0.5 (0.2-1.7)
Weiss (29)	0.6 (0.4-1.0)
Cramer (30)	0.4 (0.2-1.0)
Rosenberg (15)	0.6 (0.4-0.9)
Tzonou (20)	0.4 (0.1-1.1)
La Vecchia (18)	0.6 (0.4-1.0)
CASH (31)	0.6 (0.4-0.9)
Harlow (32)#	0.4 (0.2-0.9)
Shu (33)	1.8 (0.8-4.1)
WHO (34)	0.8 (0.6-1.0)
Booth (35)	0.5 (0.3-0.9)
Overall RR*	0.6 (0.5-0.7)

Borderline malignancy neoplasms.
* Using the method described by Prentice and Thomas (76).

ENDOMETRIAL CANCER

The hypothesis that the continuous influence of oestrogenic substances not alternated with progesterone is causally related to endometrial cancer had already been clearly formulated in the 1950s (37). At present the understanding of the basic hormonal biology of endometrial cancer is far more advanced than that of any other gynaecological malignancy. Anything that increases exposure of the endometrium to unopposed oestrogens increases the risk of the disease for the rest of a woman's life by increasing the frequency of mitosis and subsequent copying errors in the endometrium (38). Conversely, anything that decreases exposure decreases the risk (38). Reproductive factors must be considered in this framework although it must be stressed that their role in relation to endometrial cancer has received far less attention than the influence of exogenous oestrogens and obesity (39,40).

Pregnancy and fertility

Before the menopause the normal levels of oestradiol are so high that endometrial activity is stimulated to the maximum and small increases have no effect on the risk of endometrial cancer (38). What does affect the risk is change in the duration of unopposed oestrogens exposure. The endometrium of a woman with "normal" ovulatory cycles proliferates for 14 days in the cycle i.e. for some 50% of the time. During pregnancy, as well as during OC use, the time of exposure to unopposed oestrogen is reduced and this may explain the protection observed in multiparous women (38).

Nulliparous women seem to be at increased risk of endometrial cancer in most epidemiological investigations (25,39-53,89). A decrease in risk with an increasing number of chilbirths after the first one has also been reported, but less consistently (41-43,45,46,48-51,55). In some studies, however, the protective effect of parity seemed to be largely restricted to the first full-term pregnancy, risk estimates not being substantially lower with increasing numbers of births (39,52-53). In a case-control investigation conducted in the Northern part of Italy the point-estimate for nulliparity increased appreciably when allowance was made for marital status (39), suggesting that infertility and not nulliparity per se could be related to the risk of endometrial cancer. Other studies (55) however, have shown no difference or only moderately increased risk among ever-married nulliparous women.

In young women, a strong direct association between endometrial cancer and the Stein Leventhal syndrome as well as other conditions involving infertility has been shown several times (37,51). The endometrium of a woman with progesterone deficiency proliferates for considerably more than 50% of the time (38). Such a condition is very frequent in premenopausal obese women and manifests itself with amenorrhoea and irregular menstrual cycles (37).

Age at pregnancy

So far, little attention has been paid to the role of age at first and subsequent pregnancies on risk of endometrial cancer. Most epidemiological studies have shown no relation either with age at first (39,41,43,45,46,51,53) or last birth (51,53).

Recently, however, significant inverse associations with age at first and last birth emerged from a prospective investigation (55). Since, as expected, parity exerted a negative confounding effect in the relationship with age at first birth, the inverse association reached statistical significance only after adjustment for parity. This was supposed to be the reason of the discrepancy with previous studies, most of which did not present results adjusted for parity (55). Kvale et al. (55) admitted the difficulty of separating completely the effects of age at first and last births, but concluded, by analogy with what had been found for breast cancer (56), that age at every pregnancy may also have an independent effect on endometrial cancer and that low risk may derive particularly from late births.

Incomplete pregnancies showed in this prospective study (55), as well as in most previous epidemiological work, no notable association with risk of endometrial cancer.

Oral contraceptives and endometrial cancer.

There are at least six studies (27,49,57-60) which have found, with remarkable consistency in risk estimates, that OC use is associated with a significant protection against endometrial cancer. All the relative risks are close to their overall average of 0.5, indicating that OC users, on a whole, have a risk reduced by about 50% of developing endometrial cancer (Table 3).

TABLE 3: Relative risk of endometrial cancer in relation to oral contraceptive (OC) use in different studies.

Study	Relative risk (RR) in ever vs never OC users (95% confidence interval)
Weiss (57)	0.5 (0.2-1.0)
Kaufman (58)	0.4 (0.2-0.8)
Hulka (59)	0.4 (0.2-1.2)
CASH (49)	0.5 (0.3-0.8)
La Vecchia (27)	0.6 (0.2-1.3)
WHO (60)	0.5
Overall RR*	0.5 (0.3-0.5)

* Using the method described by Prentice and Thomas (76).

This protection increases with increasing duration of use, thus stressing the causal nature of the association, and appears to persist up to 10-15 years after stopping use. Since the continuous influence of oestrogenic substances unopposed by progesterone is at the present time firmly recognized as a major determinant of endometrial cancer risk (38), the protective effect of combined OCs was predictable on theoretical grounds.

Endometrial cancer, nevertheless, is a rare disease in young and middle aged women. Thus, in the absence of direct information on the possible persistence of the protection into older age, its proven impact should be considered, on a public health scale, as relatively limited.

CUTANEOUS MALIGNANT MELANOMA

Several lines of evidence have suggested a relationship between the biological behaviour of melanocytes and cutaneous malignant melanoma (CMM) and the action of female hormones. Animal experiments have shown that oestrogens and oestrogens-progestogen combinations cause an increase both in melanocyte count and in intracellular and extracellular melanin content. In human beings, proliferation of melanocyte naevi around puberty, and benign hyperpigmentation and changes in colour and size of naevi during pregnancy and during OC-use may also relate to hormonal influence (see ref 61 for a review).

Furthermore in the majority of European populations CMM incidence is consistently higher in females than in males and the only aspect in which the difference in CMM occurrence by gender is large and present in all populations is tumour location. In Caucasians, CMM except lentigo maligna melanoma (LMM), is most common on the trunk in males and lower limbs in females (61).

Menstrual and reproductive factors

Six case-control studies (62-67) attempted to measure the influence of endogenous hormones on CMM risk by assessing menstrual and reproductive factors. None of these factors seemed to have a substantial impact on risk. Age at menarche, age at menopause and duration of reproductive years did not affect CMM risk in any of the aforementioned studies.

Two investigations (63,64) showed a non-significantly elevated CMM risk (2.4 and 2.7 respectively) associated with delayed child-bearing (Table 4). A decreased risk (RR = 0.3) associated with 5 or more births was reported by Gallagher et al. (62) and Zanetti et al. (67). In the investigation by Gallagher et al. (62) a hint also emerged that surgical menopause may exert a protective effect and this finding was replicate by another study (63). The elevation of risk associated with delayed child bearing was invariably very low and non-significant (62,63,64). It was, also, claimed that superficial spreading melanoma (SSM) was the histologic type specifically influenced by female hormones. SSM cases, however, were 61 out of 87 CMM cases in the study by Holly et al. (64) and 269 out of 361 in the study by Gallagher et al. (62), rendering a meaningful differential analysis difficult (Table 4).

TABLE 4: Relative risk of melanoma by reproductive factors and type of menopause.

Study	Parity (>5 vs 0)		Age at first birth (>30 vs <25)	Type of menopause (surgical vs natural)
Holly (64)	All	1.0	2.4	0.8
	SSM	0.7	3.0	0.8
Holman (65)	All	0.7	1.0	---
	SSM	0.7	3.0	0.8
Gallagher (62)	All	0.3*	1.4	0.5*
	SSM	0.4*	1.4	0.3*
Green (63)**	All	2.3	2.7	0.4
	SSM	---	---	---
Osterlind (66)**	All	0.9	1.0	1.2
	SSM	---	---	---
Zanetti (67)**	All	0.3*#	1.0	---
	SSM	---	---	---

*   Upper 95% confidence limit < 1.0.
** Relative risk for SSM not given, but similar to all CMM.
\#   The association was weakened by adjustment for sun exposure and reaction.
SSM Superficial spreading melanoma.

The relation between infertility and CMM risk was explored in two cohort studies, one on 2575 women treated for infertility in Israel (68), and another on 2335 women treated at the Mayo Clinic in the United States (69). An increased standardized incidence ration (SIR) for melanoma was observed in the study by Ron et al. (68), (SIR = 2.0) while the SIR was only 1.2 in the study by Brinton et al. (69). If analysis is restricted to patients whose infertility was presumed to be due to progesterone deficiencey, the SIR was estimated to be 2.6 in both investigations. The similarity of the findings is interesting, but, since only 4 diagnoses of melanoma occurred in each cohort of infertile women, it is difficult to draw any conclusions.

Oral contraceptives and melanoma

The possibility that OCs may predispose women to the development of CMM was first raised in the late 1970's (70). Subsequently, at least ten case-control studies (62-67,70-73) have addressed this issue (Table 5). Three of them were conducted in North America, four in Australia, one in Great Britain, one in Denmark and one in Italy. With one exception (73), they were all population-based case-control studies. Only the first hypothesis-generating study found as association between OC use and CMM risk. All the risk estimates from subsequent studies were close to unity (between 0.7 and 1.2), thus providing evidence of the

TABLE 5: Relative risk of cutaneous malignant melanoma in relation to oral contraceptive (OC) use in different studies.

Study	Relative risk (RR) in ever vs never OC users (95% confidence interval)*
Beral (88)	1.8 (0.8-4.2)
Adam (71)	1.1 (0.7-1.8)
Bain (72)	0.8 (0.5-1.3)
Holly (64)	1.2 (0.6-2.1)
Helmrich (73)	0.8 (0.5-1.3)
Beral (70)	1.0 (0.5-1.9)
Holman (65)	1.0 (0.6-1.6)
Gallagher (62)**	1.0
Green (63)	0.7 (0.4-1.5)
Osterlind (66)	0.8 (0.6-1.1)
Zanetti (67)	1.0 (0.5-1.9)
Overall RR	0.9 (0.8-1.1)#

* () indicate confidence intervals calculated using approximate method; ** Insufficient information published to include in calculation of summary odds ratio; # p-value for test of homogeneity equal to 0.71.

98

absence of any substantial association between OCs and cutaneous malignant melanoma. The summary relative risk was 0.9, 95% confidence interval : 0.8-1.1.

In addition, three prospective studies on OC use (71,74,75) have provided some data on CMM. Thier value is, however, limited, first, because very few cases of cutaneous malignant melanoma emerged during the follow-up and, second, because such cohort studies were chiefly designed to investigate other diseases and did not include information on the most important correlates of cutaneous malignant melanoma risk. Similarly, however, to the retrospective investigations, no significant association between OC use and CMM risk emerged from a pooled analysis of cohort studies (76) and, most important, no trend of increasing risk with longer duration of use was seen.

CERVICAL CANCER

Although the epidemiology of cancer of the cervix uteri strongly suggests a sexually transmitted aetiology (2) OCs at least, among female hormones, have received great attention as agents which may themselves promote the development of such tumours. Two cohort (77,78) and six case-control studies (27,79-83) have considered dysplasias and _in situ_ neoplasias of the cervix uteri. The corresponding results, summarized in Table 6, indicate a moderately elevated relative risk among OC users: the overall relative risk (76) was above 2 (with a lower 95% confidence limit of 1.6) for cohort studies, and, though less strongly, still significantly above unity (RR = 1.3) for case-control studies as well.

In relation to invasive cervical cancer (Table 7), most published studies (three cohort (77,78,84) and five case control (27,83,85-87) found an elevated risk among OC users. The overall relative risk estimate was 1.2 for case-control studies, and in two out of three cohort studies all invasive cancers (13 and 6 respectively) were registered among pill users.

There is, therefore, a consistent series of reports indicating that OC use is associated with an increased risk of intraepithelial and invasive cervical cancer. This is further confirmed by the presence of direct duration-risk relationships in most studies. The uncertainties concerning cervical neoplasia and OCs chiefly derive from the potential confounding effects of some important risk correlates such as sexual habits and, to a lesser extent, smoking: however most recent investigations (27,85,86) have attempted to adjust for them.

Since invasive cervical cancer, on the other hand, is largely preventable through rational use of cervical

99

screening, this evidence indicates that specific attention should be paid to cervical screening from early middle age for users, or ex-users, of OCs.

TABLE 6: Relative risk of pre-invasive cervical neoplasm in relation to oral contraceptive (OC) use in different studies.

Study	Relative risk (RR) in ever vs never OC users (95% confidence interval)
Cohort studies	
Walnut Creek	5.2 (2.4-11.4)
Oxford-FPA	1.8 (1.1-2.7)
Overall RR*	2.3 (1.6-3.4)
Case-control studies	
Thomas (79)	0.9 (0.7-1.3)
Ory (80)	1.4 (1.2-1.6)
Fasal (81)	1.4 (0.4-1.3)
La Vecchia (27)	0.7 (0.4-1.1)
Molina (82)	1.2 (0.7-2.1)
Irwin (83)	1.6 (1.2-2.2)
Overall RR*	1.3 (1.2-1.5)

* Using the method described by Prentice and Thomas (76).

TABLE 7: Relative risk of invasive cervical cancer in relation to oral contraceptive (OC) use in different studies.

Study	Relative risk (RR) in ever vs never OC users (95% confidence interval)
Cohort studies	
Oxford-FPA	(13 vs 0 cases)
RCGP	2.1 (1.1-4.3)
Andolsek (84)	(6 vs 0 cases)
Case-control studies	
WHO (85)	1.2 (1.0-1.4)
Brinton (86)	1.5 (1.1-2.1)
La Vecchia (27)	1.7 (0.8-3.6)
Celentano (87)	0.7 (0.3-1.9)
Irwin (83)	0.8 (0.5-1.3)
Overall RR*	1.2 (1.0-1.4)

* Using the method described by Prentice and Thomas (76).

REFERENCES

1. WHO Prevention of cancer. (1964) Technical Report Series 276, Geneva.
2. Doll, R., and Peto, R. (1981) The causes of cancer. JNIC, 66, 1191-1308.
3. Pike, M.C. (1987) Age-related factors in cancers of the breast, ovary and endometrium. J Chron Dis, 40, 59S-69S.
4. Franceschi, S. (1989) Reproductive Factors and cancer of the breast, ovary and endometrium. Eur J Cancer Clin Oncol, 25, 1933-1943.
5. La Vecchia, C., Franceschi, S., Bruzzi, P., Parazzini, F., Boyle, P. Incidence, aetiology and prevention of adverse effects of oral contraceptives. Drug safety, in press.
6. Wynder, E.L., Dodo, H., Barber, HRK. (1969) Epidemiology of cancer of the ovary. Cancer, 23, 352-370.
7. Beral, V., Fraser, P., Chilvers, C. (1978) Does pregnancy protect against ovarian cancer ? Lancet, i, 1083-1087.
8. Weiss, N.S. (1988) Measuring the separate effects of low parity and its antecedents on the incidence of ovarian cancer. Am J Epidemiol, 128 451-455.
9. Joly, DJ, Lilienfeld, AM, Diamond, EL, Bross, IDJ. (1974) An epidemiologic study of the relationship of reproductive experience to cancer of the ovary. Am J Epidemiol, 99, 190-209.
10. Newhouse, ML, Pearson, RM, Fullerton, JM, Boesen, EA, Shannon, HS (1977) A case control study of carcinoma of the ovary. Br J Prev Soc Med, 31, 148-153.
11. Casagrande, J.T, Louie, E.W, Pike, MC, Roy, S, Ross, RK, Henderson, BE. (1979) "Incessant ovulation" and ovarian cancer. Lancet, ii, 170-173.
12. McGowan, L, Parent, L, Lednar, W, Norris, HJ. (1979) The woman at risk for developing ovarian cancer. Gynecol Oncol, 7, 325-344.
13. Hildreth, NG, Kelsey, J, Livolsi, VA et al. (1981) An epidemiologic study of epithelial carcinoma of the ovary. Am J Epidemiol, 114, 398-405.
14. Franceschi, S., La Vecchia, C., Helmrich, SP, Mangioni, C, Tognoni, G. (1982) Risk factors for epithelial ovarian cancer in Italy. Am J Epidemiol, 115, 714-719.
15. Rosenberg, L, Shapiro, S, Slone, D et al. (1982) Epithelial ovarian cancer and combination oral contraceptives. JAMA, 247, 3210-3212.
16. Cramer, DW, Hutchinson, GB, Welch, WR, Scully, RE, Ryan, KJ. (1983) Determinants of ovarian cancer risk. Reproductive experiences and family history. JNCI, 71, 711-716.
17. Rish, HA, Weiss, NS, Lyon, JL, Daling, JR, Liff, JM. (1983) Events of reproductive life and the incidence of

epithelial ovarian cancer. Am J Epidemiol, 117, 128-139.

18. La Vecchia, C, Decarli, A, Franceschi, S, Regallo, M, Tognoni, G. (1984) Age at first birth and the risk of epithelial ovarian cancer. JNCI, 73, 663-666.

19. Nasca, PC, Greenwald, P, Chorost, S, Richart, R, Caputo, T. (1984) An epidemiologic case-control study of ovarian cancer and reproductive factors. Am J Epidemiol, 119, 705-713.

20. Tzonou, A, Day, N.E, Trichopoulos, D. et al. (1984) The epidemiology of ovarian cancer in Greece: a case-control study. Eur J Cancer Clin Oncol, 20, 1045-1052.

21. Lesher, L, McGowan, L, Hartge, P, Hoover, R. (1985) Letters to the Editors: Age at first birth and risk of epithelial ovarian cancer. JNCI, 74, 1361-1362.

22. Voigt, LF, Harlow, BL, Weiss, NS. (1986) The influence of age at first birth and parity on ovarian cancer risk. Am J Epidemiol, 124, 490-491.

23. Lee, NC, Wingo, PA, Gwinn, ML et al. (1987) The reduction in risk of ovarian cancer associated with oral-contraceptive use. N Engl J Med, 316, 650-655.

24. Mori, M, Harabuchi, I, Miyake, H, Casagrande, JT, Henderson, BE, Ross, RK. (1988) Reproductive, genetic, and dietary risk factors for ovarian cancer. Am J Epidemiol, 128, 771-777.

25. Kvale, G, Heuch, I, Nissen, S, Beral, V. (1988) Reproductive factors and risk of ovarian cancer: a prospective study. Int J Cancer, 42, 246-251.

26. Wu, ML, Whittemore, AS, Paffenbarger, RS. Jr. et al. (1988) Personal and environmental characteristics related to epithelial ovarian cancer. I. Reproductive and menstrual events and oral contraceptive use. Am J Epidemiol, 128, 1216-1227.

27. La Vecchia, C, Decarli, A, Fasoli, M et al. (1986) Oral contraceptives and cancers of breast and of the female genital tract. Interim results from a case-control study. Br J Cancer, 54, 311-317.

28. Willett, WC, Bain, C, Hennekens, CH, Rosner, B, Speizer, Fe. (1981) Oral contraceptives and risk of ovarian cancer. Cancer, 48, 1684-1687.

29. Weiss, NS, Lyon, JL, Liff, JM, Vollmer, WM, Daling, JR. (1981) Incidence of ovarian cancer in relation to the use of oral contraceptives. Int J Cancer, 28, 669-671.

30. Cramer, DW, Hutchinson, GB, Welch, WR, Scully, RE, Knapp, RC. (1982) Factors affecting the association of oral contraceptives and ovarian cancer. N Engl J Med, 307, 1047.

31. The Cancer and Steroid Hormone Study of the Centers for Disease Control and the National Institute of Child Health and Human Development. (1987) The reduction in risk of ovarian cancer associated with oral-contraceptive use. N Engl J Med, 316, 650-655.

32. Harlow, BL, Weiss, NS, Roth, GJ, Chu, J. and Daling, JR. (1988) Case-control study of borderline ovarian tumors: reproductive history and exposure to exogenous female hormones. Cancer Res, 48, 5849-5852.

33. Shu, X.O., Dunham, LJ, Casper, J. et al. (1966) Epidemiology of cancers of uterine cervix and corpus, breast and ovary in Israel and New York City. JNCI, 37, 1-95.

34. WHO Collaborative Study of Neoplasia and Steroid Contraceptives. (1989) Epithelial ovarian cancer and combined oral contraceptives. Int J Epidemiol, 18, 538-545.

35. Booth, M, Beral, V, Smith, P. (1989) Risk factors for ovarian cancer: a case-control study. Br J Cancer, 60, 592-598.

36. Fathalla, MF. (1972) Factors in the causation and incidence of ovarian cancer. Obstet Gynecol Surv, 27, 751-768.

37. De Waard, F. (1958) On the aethiology of endometrial carcinoma. Acta Endocrinol, 29, 279-294.

38. Key, TJA, Pike, MC. (1988) The dose-effect relationship between 'unopposed' oestrogens and endometrial mitotic rate: its central role in explaining and predicting endometrial cancer risk. Br J Cancer, 57, 205-212.

39. La Vecchia, C, Franceschi, S, Decarli, A, Gallus, G, Tognoni, G. (1984) Risk factors for endometrial cancer at different ages. JNCI, 73, 667-671.

40. Ziel, H.K., Finkle, W.D. (1975) Increased risk of endometrial carcinoma among users of conjugated estrogens. N Engl J Med, 293, 1167-1170.

41. Stewart, HL, Dunham, LJ, Casper, J. et al. (1966) Epidemiology of cancers of uterine cervix and corpus, breast and ovary in Isreal and New York City. JNCI, 37, 1-95.

42. Dunn, LJ, Bradbury, JT. (1967) Endocrine factors in endometrial carcinoma. Am J Obstet Gynecol, 97, 465-471.

43. Elwood, JM, Cole, P, Rothman, KJ, Kaplan, SD. (1977) Epidemiology of endometrial cancer. JNCI, 59, 1055-1060.

44. McDonald, TW, Annegers, JF, O'Fallon, WM, Dockerty, MB, Malkasian ,GD, Kurlan, LT. (1977) Exogenous estrogen and endometrial carcinoma: case-control and incidence study. Am J Obstet Gynecol, 127, 572-580.

45. Miller, AB, Barclay, THC, Choi, NW et al. (1980) A study of cancer, parity and age at first pregnancy. J Chron Dis, 33, 595-605.

46. Kelsey, JL, LiVolsi, VA, Holford, TR et al. (1982) A case-control study of cancer of the endometrium. Am J Epidemiol, 116, 333-342.

47. Beral, V. (1985) Long term effects of childbearing on health. J Epidemiol Commun Health, 39, 343-346.

48. Pettersson, B, Adami, HO, Bergstrom, R, Jahansson, EDB. (1986) Menstrula span - a time-limited risk factors for endometrial carcinoma. Acta Obstet Gynecol Scand, 65, 247-255.

49. The Cancer Steroid Hormone Study of the Centers for Disease Control and the National Institute of Child Health and Human Development. (1987) Combination oral contraceptive use and the risk of endometrial cancer. JAMA, 257, 796-800.

50. Plesko, I, Preston-Martin, S, Day, NE, Tzonou, A, Dimitrova, E, Somogy, J. (1985) Parity and cancer risk in Slovakia. Int J Cancer, 36, 529-533.

51. Henderson, BE, Casagrande, JT, Pike, MC, Mack, T, Rosario, I, Duke, A. (1983) The epidemiology of endometrial cancer in young women. Br J Cancer, 47, 749-756.

52. Salmi, T. (1979) Risk factors in endometrial carcinoma with special reference to the use of estrogens. Acta Obstet Gynecol Scand, 86 Suppl, 1-119.

53. Wynder, E.L., Escher, G.C., Mantel, N. (1966) An epidemiological investigation of cancer of the endometrium. Cancer, 19, 489-520.

54. Logan, W. P.D. (1953) Marriage and childbearing in relation to cancer of the breast and uterus. Lancett ii, 1199-1202.

55. Kvale, G, Heuch, I, Ursin, G. (1988) Reproductive factors and risk of cancer of the uterine corpus: a prospective study. Cancer Res, 48, 6217-6221.

56. Kvale, G, Heuch, I. (1987) A prospective study of reproductive factors and breast cancer. II. Age at first and last birth. Am J Epidemiol, 126, 842-850.

57. Weiss, NS, Sayvetz, TA. (1980) Incidence of endometrial cancer in relation to the use of oral contraceptive. N Engl J Med, 302, 551-554.

58. Kaufman, DW, Shapiro, S, Slone, D, Rosenberg, L, Miettined, OS et al. (1980) Decreased risk of endometrial cancer among oral-contraceptive users. N Engl J Med, 303, 1045-1047.

59. Hulka, BS, Chambless, LE, Kaufman, DG, Fowler, WC Jr, Greenberg, BG. (1982) Protection against endometrial carcinoma by combination-product oral contraceptives. JAMA, 259, 475-477.

60. Who (1988) Collaborative Study of Neoplasia and Steroid Contraceptives, Endometrial cancer and combined oral contraceptives. Int J Epidemiol, 17, 263-269.

61. Franceschi, S., Baron, A.E., La Vecchia, C. The influence of female hormones on malignant melanoma. Tumori, in press.

62. Gallagher, RP, Elwood, JM, Hill, GB, Coldman,AJ, Threfall, WJ, Spinelli, JJ. (1985) Reproductive factors, oral contraceptives and risk of malignant melanoma:

Western Canada melanoma study. Br J Cancer, 52, 901-907.

63. Green, A., Bain, C. (1985) Hormonal factors and melanoma in women. Med J Aust, 142, 446-448.

64. Holly, EA, Weiss, NS, Liff, JM. (1983) Cutaneous melanoma in relation to exogenous hormones and reproductive factors. JNCI, 70, 827-831.

65. Holman, CDJ, Armstrong, BK, Heenan, PJ. (1984) Cutaneous malignant melanoma in women: exogenous sex hormones and reproductive factors. Br J Cancer, 50, 673-680.

66. Osterlind, A, Tucker, MA, Stone, BJ, Jensen, OM. (1988) The Danish case-control study of cutaneous malignant melanoma. III. Hormonal and reproductive factors in women. Int J Cancer, 42, 821-824.

67. Zanetti, R, Franceschi, S, Rosso, S, Bidoli, E, Colonna, S. Cutaneous malignant melanoma in females: the role of hormonal and reproductive factors. Int J Epidemiol, in press.

68. Ron, E, Lunenfeld, B, Menczer, J, Blumstein, T, Katz, L, Oelsner, G, Serr, D. (1987) Cancer incidence in a cohort of infertile women. Am J Epidemiol, 125, 780-790.

69. Brinton, LA, Melton, LJ.III, Malkasian, GD, Bond, A, hoover, R. (1989) Cancer risk after evaluation for infertility. Am J Epidemiol, 129, 712-722.

70. Beral, V, Evans, S, Shaw, H, Milton, G. (1984) Oral contraceptive use and malignant melanoma in Australia. Br J Cancer, 50, 681-685.

71. Adam, SA, Sheaves, JK, Wright, NH, Mosser, G, Harris, RW, Vessey, MP. (1981) A case-control study of the possible association between oral contraceptives and malignant melanoma. Br J Cancer, 44, 45-50.

72. Bain, C, Hennekens, CH, Speizer, FE, Rosner, B, Willet, W, Belanger, C. (1982) Oral contraceptive use and malignant melanoma. JNCI, 68, 537-539.

73. Helmrich, SP, Rosenberg, L, Kaufman, DW, Miller, DR, Schottenfeld, D, Stolley, PD, Shapiro, S. (1984) Lack of an elevated risk of malignant melanoma in relation to oral contraceptive use. JNCI, 72, 617-620.

74. Kay, C.R. (1981) Malignant melanoma and oral contraceptives. Br J Cancer, 44, 479.

75. Ramcharan, S, Pellegrin, FA, Ray, R, Hsu, JP. (1981) A prospective study of the side effects of oral contraceptives. The Walnut Creek contraceptive study. Vol. III, NIH Publication No. 81-564, Bethesda MD.

76. Prentice, RL, Thomas, DB. (1987) On the epidemiology of oral contraceptives and disease. (1987) Advances in cancer research, 49, 285-401, Academic Press.

77. Royal College of General Practitioners. (1974) Oral contraceptive and health. An interim report from the Oral Contraception Study of the Royal College of general Practitioners. Pitman Medical, London.

78. Vessey, M, Doll, R, Peto, R, Johson, B, Viggins, P.

(1976) A long-term following-up study of women using different methods of contraception - an interim report. J Biosoc Sci, 8, 373-427.

79. Thomas, DB. (1972) Relationship of oral contraceptives to cervical carcinogenesis. Obstet Gynecol, 40, 508-518.

80. Ory, HW, Conger, SB, Naib, Z, Tyler, CW Jr, Hatcher, RA. (1977) Preliminary analysis of oral contraceptive use and risk of developing premalignant lesion of the uterine cervix. in: Garattini and Gerendes (Eds) Pharmacology of steroid contraceptive drugs, pp. 211-224, Raven Press, New York.

81. Fasal, E, Simmons, ME, Kampert, JB. (1981) Factors associated with high and low risk of cervical neoplasia. JNCI, 66, 631-636.

82. Molina, R, Thomas, DB, Dabances, A, Lopez, J, Ray, RM, et al. (1988) Oral contraceptives and cervical carcinoma in situ in Chile. Cancer Res, 48, 1011-1015.

83. Irwin, KL, Rosero-Bixby, L, Oberle, MW, Lee, NC, Whatley, AS et al. (1988) Oral contraceptives and oral cancer risk in Costa Rica. Detection bias or causal association ? JAMA, 259, 59-64.

84. Andolsek, L, Kovacic, U, Kozuh, M, Litt, B. (1983) Oral contraceptives and cervical cancer. Lancet, ii, 1310.

85. WHO (1985) collaborative Study of Neoplasia and Steroid Contraceptives. Invasive cervical cancer and combined oral contraceptives. Int J Epidemiol, 17, 263-269.

86. Brinton, La, Huggins, GR, Lehman, HF, Mallin, K, Savitz, DA et al. (1986) Long-term use of oral contraceptives and risk of invasive cervical cancer. Int J Cancer, 38, 339-344.

87. Celentano, DD, Klassen, AC, Weisman, CS, Rosenshein, NB. (1987) The role of contraceptive use in cervical cancer: the Maryland cervical cancer case-control study. Am J Epidemiol, 126, 592-604.

88. Beral, V, Ramcharan, S, Faris, R. (1977) Malignant and oral contraceptive use among women in California. Br J Cancer, 36, 804-809.

89. Fox, H, Sen, DK. (1970) A controlled study of the constitutional stigmata of endometrial adenocarcinoma. Br J Cancer, 24, 30-36.

9

TOBACCO-SPECIFIC NITROSAMINES: UNDERESTIMATED CARCINOGENS IN TOBACCO AND TOBACCO SMOKE

Sophia Fisher, Bertold Spiegelhalder and Rudolf Preussmann
Institute for Toxicology and Chemotherapy, German Cancer Research Center, Im Neuenheimer Feld 280, 6900 Heidelberg, Germany

INTRODUCTION

Smoking is causally related to the occurrence of cancer of the oral cavity, larynx, lung and oesophagus. It is also a contributory factor to the development of cancer of the pancreas, kidney and urinary bladder (1). Tobacco smoke contains more than 3800 compounds (2). Some of these compounds such as the polynuclear aromatic hydrocarbons (PAH), aromatic amines, N-nitroso compounds, polonium-210 and others are known to be strong carcinogens. There are also toxic smoke constituents such as nicotine, carbon monoxide, nitrogen oxide, hydrogen cyanide and others (1).

The tobacco specific nitrosamines (TSNA*) are derived from the alkaloids of the tobacco plant (Figure 1). By nitrosation of the tertiary amine nicotine, the main alkaloid, two nitrosamines can be formed: 4-(Methylnitrosamino)-1-(3-pyridyl)-1-butanone (NNK) and N'-nitrosonornicotine (NNN). NNN can also be formed by nitrosation of the secondary amine nornicotine, a minor alkaloid of tobacco. Nitrosation of the secondary amines anatabine and anabasine, both minor alkaloids of tobacco,

---

* The abbreviations used and the chemical substance prime names according to Chemical Abstracts in brackets are: TSNA, tobacco-specific nitrosamines; NNN, N'-nitrosonornicotine, (3-(1-nitroso-2-pyrrolidinyl)-pyridine); NNK, 4-(methylnitrosamino)-1-(3-pyridyl)-1-butanone; NAB, N'-nitrosoanabasine, (3-(1-nitroso-2-piperidinyl)-pyridine); NAT, N'-nitrosoanatabine, (1,2,3,6-tetrahydro-1-nitroso-2,3'-bipyridine); PHA, polynuclear aromatic hydrocarbons; B(a)P, benzo(a)pyren.

TABLE 1: Carcinogenicity of tobacco-specific nitrosamines (3)

Nitrosamine	Species and strains	Route of application	Principal target organ	Dose
NNN	A/J mouse	i.p.	Lung	21.2 mg/mouse
	F344 rat	s.c.	Nasal cavity, esophagus	35.4-601.8 mg/rat
		p.o.	Esophagus, nasal cavity	177.2-637.9 mg/rat
	Sprague-Dawley rat	p.o.	Nasal cavity	1559.4 mg/rat
	Syrian golden hamsters	s.c.	Trachea, nasal cavity	159.5-372.1 mg/hamster
NNK	A/J mouse	i.p.	Lung	25.9 mg/mouse
	F344 rat	s.c.	Nasal cavity, lung, liver	41.4-580.2 mg/rat
	Syrian golden hamster	s.c.	Trachea, lung, nasal cavity	186.5 mg/hamster 1.0 mg/hamster
NAT	F344 rat	s.c.	none	37.8-529.8 mg/rat
NAB	F344 rat	p.o.	Esophagus	573.6-2294.4 mg/rat
	Syrian golden hamster	s.c.	none	382.4 mg/hamster

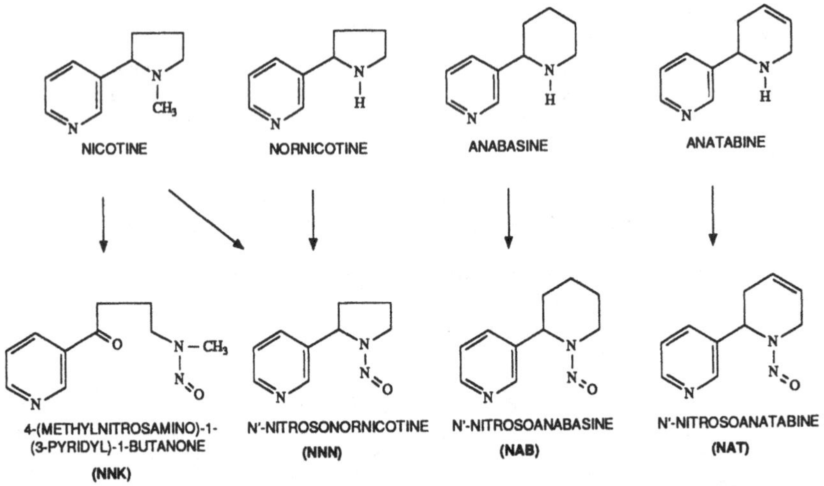

Figure 1: Structure formulas of the tobacco alkaloids and the corresponding TSNA.

leads to the formation of N'-nitrosoanabasine (NAB) and N'-nitrosoanatabine (NAT) (3,4). The TSNA have been found in tobacco and in tobacco smoke in high concentrations (3,5-7).

NNN and NNK are potent and organ-specific carcinogens. They induce benign and malignant tumors in mice, rats and hamsters (Table 1) (3,8). Upon s.c. injection, NNN induces primarily papilloma and carcinoma of the nasal cavity but also oesophageal tumors at doses down to 35.4 mg/rat, i.e. 17.7 mg/kg. Administration of NNN in the drinking water to rats causes benign and malignant tumors of the oesophagus in addition to nasal cavity tumors (3). These results indicate, that the organospecificity of NNN depends on the route of administration (3). NNK is the most potent carcinogen among the TSNA. It induces lung tumors in mice; nasal cavity, lung and liver tumors in rats; and nasal cavity, tracheal, and lung tumors in hamsters. The most important observation is the induction of lung adenomas and adenocarcinomas in hamsters in response to doses of 1mg/hamster, and squamous carcinoma and adenocarcinoma of the lung in rats at doses of 41.4 mg/rat (3). Furthermore NNK has the potential to exert a local carcinogenic effect. Upon topical application to SENCAR mice of 5.8 mg NNK per mouse, NNK induced skin tumors with an incidence of 79% and lung adenomas with an incidence of 59% (9). The organospecificity of NNK for the lung is striking (8). NAB is a weak carcinogen, and NAT appears not to be carcinogenic (3).

The amount of tar in cigarette smoke is widely accepted as an index of the biological activity and the carcinogenic potential of cigarette smoke (1). In the Federal Republic of Germany as in many other European countries the tar and nicotine deliveries have to be declared (10) to give the consumer an orientation on the relative risk associated with the individual brands. A legislative regulation for the countries of the European Community to reduce the tar deliveries has been passed recently. An upper limit of 15 mg tar per cigarette from 1993 and a further reduction to 12 mg tar per cigarette from 1996 has been decided (11). During the last few years cigarette manufacturers have reduced tar and nicotine deliveries to approach so called "safer cigarettes" (1,12). In addition, a new class of cigarettes with very low tar has become increasingly important in consumption. A suitable index for the carcinogenic potential of cigarette smoke should represent the amount of the major carcinogens in mainstream smoke, i.e. the tar delivery should also give an orientation on the amount of the strong carcinogens NNN and NNK in mainstream smoke.

TSNA IN COMMERCIAL CIGARETTES

In a representative study more than 170 different cigarette brands from several European countries and the USA have been analyzed for TSNA in tobacco and in mainstream smoke as well as for nitrate in tobacco. For the study a large variety of cigarettes has been chosen. There were filter and non filter cigarettes with very high, high, moderate, low and very low tar and nicotine deliveries. The classification of cigarettes on the basis of their tar deliveries according to IARC is shown in Table 2.

TABLE 2: Classification of cigarettes on the basis of their tar yields according to IARC (1).

Description of yield	Tar yield (mg/cigarette)
very low	< 4.9
low	5-9.9
moderate	10-14.9
high	15-20
very high	20 and over

The tar and nicotine deliveries are correlated. For most cigarettes a relatively constant ratio of about 15:1 for tar to nicotine is valid. For a few cigarettes this ratio has recently been changed to about 10:1 (13).
The ranges for the TSNA concentrations in tobacco and in mainstream smoke as well as the ranges for the nitrate levels of the investigated cigarettes are presented in Table 3, together with the corresponding ranges for the declared tar and nicotine deliveries. NNN in mainstream smoke ranged from 5 ng/cigarette up to 1353 ng/cigarette, NNK values from not detectable to 1749 ng/cigarette. For preformed TSNA in tobacco the observed range for NNN was from 50 to 12454 ng/cigarette and for NNK from not detectable to 10745 ng/cigarette. The nitrate levels were between 0.6 and 19.4 mg/cigarette. For the cigarettes of most countries high as well as low TSNA and nitrate levels could be found. Extremely high TSNA concentrations were determined for few Italian nonfilter cigarettes. Very high TSNA concentrations were also observed for nonfilter cigarettes made of dark tobaccos which have been bought in West Germany and France. The lowest TSNA concentrations were found in nonfilter Oriental type cigarettes on the West German market (14,7). With the exception of the dark tobacco type cigarettes, which are generally high in TSNA (14,15), and few specific

110

TABLE 3: Ranges for tar, nicotine and TSNA deliveries in mainstream smoke as well as concentrations for preformed TSNA and nitrate in tobacco for commercial cigarettes from several European countries and the USA (7).

Country	Tar mg/cig min-max	Nicotine mg/cig min-max	NNN ng/cig MS min-max	NNN ng/cig Tobacco min-max	NNK ng/cig MS min-max	NNK ng/cig Tobacco min-max	NO_3^- mg/cig min-max	n
Austria	9- 15	0.7- 0.9	42- 172	306- 1122	12- 100	92- 310	4.2- 8.0	5
Belgium	13- 16	1.0- 1.3	38- 203	504- 1939	29- 150	219- 594	1.8- 10.8	7
FRG	1- 28	0.1- 2.0	5- 625	50- 5316	n.d.- 432	n.d.- 1120	0.6- 14.4	55
France	6- 44	0.3- 2.7	11- 1000	120- 6019	19- 498	57- 990	1.5- 19.4	20
Great Britain	lt- mt	n.a.	17- 123	140- 1218	18- 103	92- 433	1.4- 8.0	12
Italy	n.a.	n.a.	21- 1353	632- 12454	8- 1749	153-10745	6.2- 13.3	10
Netherlands	1- 18	0.2- 1.5	9- 163	58- 1647	5- 102	105- 587	1.5- 8.8	19
Poland	n.a.	n.a.	121- 347	870- 2760	38- 105	140- 450	4.4- 12.8	6
Sweden	9- 23	0.8- 1.8	44- 141	544- 1511	27- 84	192- 569	2.4- 8.6	10
Switzerland	12- 15	0.9- 1.2	121- 226	1280- 2208	69- 124	450- 554	6.4- 7.8	3
USA	n.a.	n.a.	54- 197	993- 1947	41- 145	433- 733	6.2- 13.5	20
USSR	n.a.	n.a.	23- 312	60- 850	4- 40	n.d.- 150	1.7- 9.1	9

MS=mainstream smoke; n.d.=not detected (MS: <4ng/cigarette, tobacco: <50 ng/cigarette); n.a.= not available; lt=low tar; mt=middle tar; n= number of cigarette brands analyzed, FRG = Federal Republic of Germany..

Italian nonfilter cigarettes the TSNA levels of the cigarette brands from the different countries generally were in a similar range. More than 90 % of the cigarettes showed mainstream smoke concentrations below 300 ng/cigarette NNN and 200 ng/cigarette NNK. The mainstream smoke concentrations of the strong carcinogens NNN and NNK are higher than the mainstream smoke concentration of the strong carcinogen benzo(a)pyren (B(a)P), the representative compound for the polynuclear aromatic hydrocarbons. The B(a)P mainstream smoke concentration is between 5 and 78 ng/cigarette (1). Thus the TSNA are the most abundant carcinogens found in mainstream smoke.

It is not possible to attribute a certain TSNA level to a specific cigarette brand as it is the case for tar and nicotine (14). Cigarettes of the same brand of different production batches might show different TSNA levels as it is shown in Table 4 for a blend filter cigarette with moderate tar and nicotine yields and for a nonfilter cigarette made of dark tobaccos with high tar and nicotine yields. Differences in the TSNA mainstream smoke concentrations of more than a factor of 2 could be demonstrated (14). Furthermore, individual brands exhibited differences in the TSNA concentration. For the same two very popular cigarette brands, a blend filter and an American-blend filter cigarette, with moderate tar and nicotine delivery,

111

TABLE 4:   Dependency of TSNA levels   on the production batch
(14)

Cigarette   NNN   NNK
                                          (ng/cig)* (ng/cig)*

West German blend filter cigarette A   130   78
West German blend filter cigarette B   85   55

West German dark nonfilter cigarette A   625   432
West German dark nonfilter cigarette B   674   333
West German dark nonfilter cigarette C   620   290
West German dark nonfilter cigarette D   270   185

A,B,C,D: Different production batches, * mainstream smoke
concentration.

purchased in 8 different countries differences in TSNA
delivery by about a factor of 2 and more could be observed
as is shown in Table 5 (7). These results demonstrated that
the actual tobacco composition is responsible for the TSNA
yields in mainstream smoke.

TABLE 5: Comparison of TSNA deliveries in mainstream smoke
for the same very popular cigarette brands purchased in
different countries (7).

| | Blend filter cigarette | | American-blend filter cigarette | |
	NNN (ng/cig)	NNK (ng/cig)	NNN (ng/cig)	NNK (ng/cig)
Austria	159	100	172	98
Belgium	90	70	128	93
FRG*	146	88	179	145
France	121	68	230	146
Great Britain	85	60	123	90
The Netherlands	126	77	163	102
Sweden	-	-	86	54
Switzerland	127	69	-	-
USA	125	112	143	121

----
*FRG= Federal Republic of Germany

PARAMETER FOR THE CARCINOGENIC POTENTIAL OF CIGARETTE SMOKE

To check whether the tar delivery is a suitable index for
the carcinogenic potential of cigarette smoke the NNN and

NNK deliveries in mainstream smoke of the investigated cigarettes were related to their declared tar deliveries, but no correlation could be observed (7). The calculated linear correlation coefficient are: NNN/tar: $r^2=0.23$; NNK/tar: $r^2=0.22$. The poor linear correlation coefficients indicate that cigarettes with low tar deliveries might have much higher TSNA deliveries than cigarettes with higher tar deliveries, or cigarettes with the same tar yield might have very different TSNA deliveries and high tar cigarettes might have very low TSNA concentrations in mainstream smoke (14,7). This does not mean that high tar cigarettes are not hazardous. It has been proven that the reduction of tar of more than 20 mg/cigarette in the sixties to 10-15 mg/cigarette nowadays has drastically decreased the risk for lung cancer (12). But it has to be emphasized that there are drastic differences in the TSNA delivery of cigarettes and that some of the so called "less harmful" cigarettes deliver high amounts of the strong carcinogens NNN and NNK.

Tar and TSNA are **independent** smoke constituents. The tar delivery is not a sufficient parameter for the carcinogenic potential of cigarette smoke, since it does not represent the amount of the strong carcinogens NNN and NNK, which are present in mainstream smoke in high concentrations. Despite the fact that there is presently no experimental model available to elucidate the contribution of the individual carcinogenic compounds such as PAH, TSNA, aromatic amines and others, the tar delivery alone, although crucial as it is representative of the amount of PAH and related compounds, seems not to represent sufficiently the risk associated with smoking, especially not for cigarettes with moderate to very low tar yields. To represent the carcinogenic potential of cigarette smoke sufficiently at least the major carcinogens in mainstream smoke, the TSNA, should be determined and declared by an additional and adequate parameter (14,7).

PREFORMED TSNA IN TOBACCO-INFLUENCE OF NITRATE AND TOBACCO TYPE

TSNA are formed during curing and fermentation of tobacco by nitrosation of the tobacco alkaloids. The nitrosating agent is nitrite which is formed by microbial reduction of nitrate (16). Fresh green tobacco leaves do not contain TSNA (16; B. Spiegelhalder et al., unpublished data).

The nitrate content of tobacco seems to be the main influencing factor for the amount of preformed TSNA in tobacco (6). The correlation between the nitrate content and the amount of preformed NNN and NNK in tobacco for West German cigarettes is shown in Figure 2. It has to be noted

113

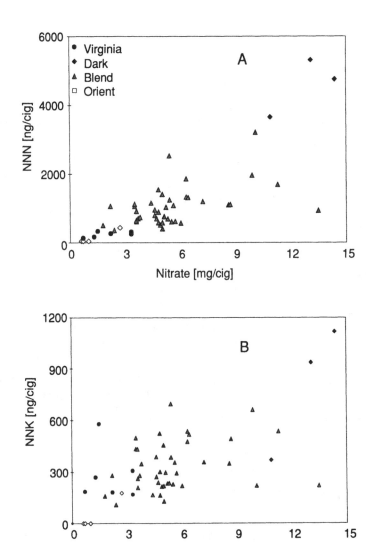

Figure 2: Dependence of the level of preformed NNN and NNK in tobacco on the nitrate content for commercial West German cigarettes (A = NNN, B = NNK) (6).

that the nitrate content of the final product has been
determined, which is just a vague parameter for the nitrate
content after harvesting and which does not represent the
nitrite content during post-harvest processing. But nitrite
is the actual nitrosating agent. The correlation for NNK is
not as good as for NNN (NNK/nitrate: r^2 = 0.61; NNK/nitrate:
r^2 = 0.40). Further factors, especially the tobacco type
seem to have an additional influence on NNK formation (6).
    There are three main tobacco types: Burley tobaccos,
which generally have a high nitrate content and which are
air-cured but protected from direct sun-light, Oriental
tobaccos, which generally have a low nitrate content and
which are sun-cured and the low nitrate Virginia tobaccos,
which are flue-cured (17).
    To investigate the influence of the tobacco type on the
TSNA level several cut and powdered tobacco samples from
pure tobacco types have been analyzed for TSNA and nitrate
(6). The results are presented in Table 6.

TABLE 6: TSNA and nitrate levels of several pure tobacco
types (6).

	NNN (ppb)		NNK (ppb)		NO_3^- (%)		n
Burley	1300-	8850	100-	1400	1.0-	4.1	8
Oriental	20-	460	n.n.-	70	0.02-	0.60	10
Virginia	10-	600	30-	1100	traces-	0.30	8

The highest TSNA levels were found in Burley tobaccos, which
are high in nitrate. High TSNA levels can also be found in
the nitrate rich stems of the various tobacco types. The
lowest TSNA levels were determined in Oriental type tobaccos
which have a low nitrate level. The low nitrate Virginia
type tobaccos also showed low levels of preformed TSNA but
in contrast to the other tobacco types NNK levels equalled
or mostly exceeded NNN levels. This phenomenon might be
caused by the different post-harvest processing of Virginia
tobacco. In blend cigarettes, which are a mixture of
Burley, Oriental, Virginia and other tobacco types, TSNA
levels increased with increasing nitrate level. The
proportion of Virginia tobaccos is the main cause for a
higher NNK level in relation to their nitrate content. Thus
the actual tobacco composition of the blends is the main
factor responsible for the TSNA level (6).

ORIGIN OF TSNA IN MAINSTREAM SMOKE

The TSNA level in mainstream smoke is predominantly
influenced by the amount of preformed TSNA in tobacco which

115

are transferred into the mainstream smoke to a certain degree during smoking. Formation of NNN and NNK from nicotine during smoking (pyrosynthesis) does not occur (18). To verify that a pyrosynthesis does not occur the TSNA precursors nitrate and nicotine were added to the cigarettes prior to smoking. The mainstream smoke concentration of NNN and NNK was not significantly changed, whereas nitrate addition resulted in an increase of NAB and NAT, which can be explained by the much easier nitrosation of secondary amines. The nitrate spiking level was between 4 and 20 mg/cigarette, whereas for the cigarettes investigated the original nitrate level was mostly below 10 mg/cigarette (18,6). The nicotine spiking level was 10 mg/cigarette, which is about the nicotine content of commercial cigarettes with moderate nicotine deliveries (18; data received from Forschungsgesellschaft Rauchen und Gesundheit, Hamburg, FRG).

Furthermore, for the cigarettes investigated, the relationship between the mainstream smoke concentration and the level of preformed NNN and NNK in tobacco was constant and did not depend on the level of the NNN and NNK precursors in tobacco, neither on nitrate nor on nicotine (18). The dependencies of the mainstream smoke/tobacco-ratios for NNN and NNK on the smoke nicotine level and the nitrate content of the tobacco for West German nonfilter cigarettes are graphically presented in Figure 3 and 4. The smoke nicotine level of nonfilter cigarettes can be considered, roughly, to represent the amount of nicotine in tobacco since the transfer rate for nicotine is relatively constant for nonfilter cigarettes (18). Since the cigarettes were different in size, the mainstream smoke/tobacco-ratios have been corrected for the cigarettes lenghts. Furthermore, for the dependence of the mainstream smoke/tobacco-ratios on the nitrate level of tobacco the ratios have additionally been corrected for the ventilation ratio (18). Ventilation causes a smaller proportion of the puff volume to be drawn through the pyrolysis zone and thus the mainstream smoke is diluted with air according to the ventilation ratio (1). In the case of nonfilter cigarettes some ventilation can be achieved by permeation of air through the cigarette paper, i.e. the ventilation is dependent on the porosity of the paper (1). For filter cigarettes more ventilation can be achieved by perforated filter tips (1). As can be seen in Figure 3 and 4 the scattering of the datapoints for NNK is higher than for NNN. No dependence on the nicotine yield could be observed. The mainstream smoke/tobacco ratios were also independent of the nitrate level with few exceptions for NNK. The nitrate-rich dark tobacco type cigarettes show much higher mainstream smoke/tobacco ratios for NNK than all other cigarettes (18).

At the moment it is not known whether the different

116

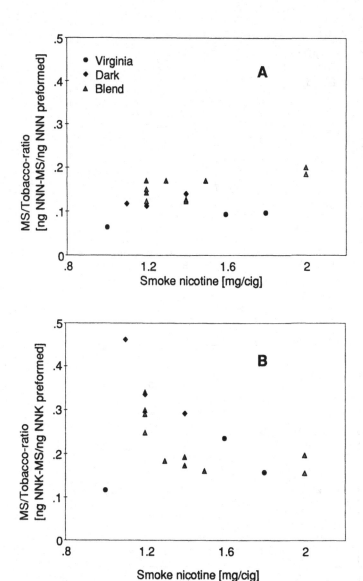

Figure 3: Dependence of the mainstream smoke/tobacco-ratios (MS/Tobacco-ratios) for NNN and NNK on the nicotine delivery for West German nonfilter cigarettes. The ratios have been corrected for the different cigarette lenghts (A = NNN, B = NNK) (18).

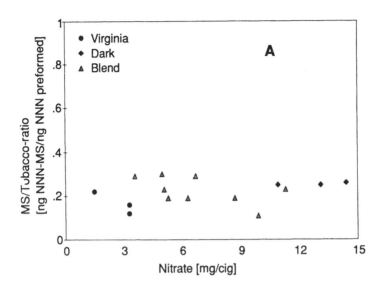

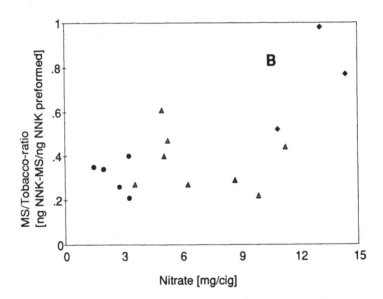

Figure 4: Dependence of the mainstream smoke/tobacco-ratios (MS/Tobacco-ratios) for NNN and NNK on the nitrate level of the tobacco. The ratios have been corrected for the different cigarette lenghts and the different ventilation ratios (A = NNN, B = NNK) (18).

behaviour of dark tobacco type cigarettes with respect to NNK is due to the tobacco type or the very high nitrate content. For these types of cigarettes a synthesis of NNK during the smoking procedure can not be excluded. But in general the dark tobacco type cigarettes do not play an important role in total tobacco consumption (13,19). Thus with the exception of NNK in dark tobaco type cigarettes the level of NNN and NNK in mainstream smoke can only be attributed to the transfer of these nitrosamines from tobacco (18).

INFLUENCE OF SMOKING BEHAVIOUR ON THE TSNA MAINSTREAM SMOKE CONCENTRATION

The transfer of TSNA from tobacco into the mainstream smoke is influenced by the total volume drawn through the cigarette during smoking, which is dependent on the puff volume and the puff frequency (20).

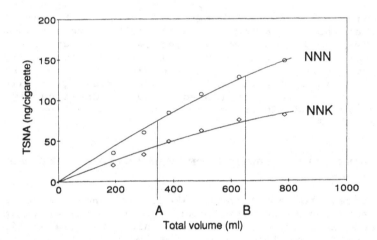

Figure 5: Dependence of the NNN and NNK concentration in mainstream smoke on the total volume drawn through a cigarette during smoking (20).
A = average inhalation volume of smokers when smoking moderate tar/moderate nicotine cigarettes (22)
B = average inhalation volume of smokers when smoking low tar/low nicotine cigarettes (22).

As is shown in Figure 5 for a low tar/low nicotine cigarette the TSNA concentration in mainstream smoke increases with increasing total volume. The smoking behaviour of smokers is mainly influenced by the nicotine delivery, since nicotine intake is the major reason for smoking. To maintain an adequate nicotine intake when low nicotine cigarettes are smoked, smokers inhale with a higher puff volume and more often, which means with a higher total inhalation volume (21,22), and consequently in a higher TSNA intake.

According to the results of Puustinen et al. (22) the total inhalation volume of smokers in the case of moderate tar/moderate nicotine cigarettes is 345 ml as compared to 650 ml in the case of low tar/low nicotine cigarettes. For the normally applied standard smoking conditions for mainstream smoke analyses a total volume of 300 ml is achieved, which is rather close to the inhalation volume for moderate yield cigarettes (20). For the same amount of preformed TSNA in tobacco the smoker of a low nicotine cigarette (which is represented by B in Figure 5) has almost twice the TSNA intake of the smoker of a moderate nicotine cigarette (which is represented by A). Presumably this finding is also true for tar and other hazardous smoke constituents, i.e. that low yield cigarettes can not always be considered to be less harmful. It has to be emphasized again that the risk associated with high and very high yield cigarettes should not be underestimated. But for risk evaluation of low nicotine cigarettes, especially in comparison to moderate nicotine cigarettes, the increased intake of smoke constituents with increasing inhalation volume has to be considered (20). Consequently low NNN/nicotine and NNK/nicotine ratios would mean a low exposure to TSNA.

APPROACHING THE REDUCTION OF CARCINOGENIC COMPOUNDS IN CIGARETTE SMOKE

One approach to reduce the intake of carcinogenic compounds by smokers and to develop "less harmful" cigarettes is the simultaneous reduction of tar and nicotine yields (1,12). As discussed above this concept has to be questionned due to the increased intake of smoke constituents with increasing inhalation volume. Another approach to develop "less harmful" cigarettes is an increase of the nicotine in relation to the tar delivery, since nicotine is the major reason for smoking and smokers' interest is to maintain an adequate nicotine intake (23,24). A relative increase in nicotine would result in a decreased total inhalation volume and thus the intake of TSNA and other smoke constituents as e.g. tar would be reduced. A nicotine delivery of about 0.8 to 1.0 mg/cigarette, which is the nicotine delivery of the most popular cigarettes (13), and a tar delivery of around 4 mg/cigarette might be suitable. This concept had so far been rejected due to synthesis of NNN and NNK during the smoking procedure postulated by Hoffmann and co-workers (25,26). But according to our results a pyrosynthesis does not occur and therefore, with an increase of the nicotine delivery in relation to tar, smokers intake of nicotine could be maintained and the intake of tar decreased without increasing the mainstream smoke concentration of the strong carcinogens NNN and NNK (18).

AVERAGE TSNA INTAKE BY SMOKERS

TABLE 7: Average TSNA exposure situation of smokers in different countries. The data are calculated on the basis of the average mainstream smoke concentration of the three most popular cigarette brands in each country and a daily consumption of 20 cigarettes (7).

Country	NNN (ug/day)	NNK (µg/day)
Federal Republic of Germany	3.0	2.0
Great Britain	0.5	1.0
Poland	5.0	1.0
Sweden	1.0	1.0
USA	3.0	2.0

Table 7 presents the daily average exposure situation to TSNA for smokers of different countries. To calculate these values the TSNA levels of the 3 most popular cigarette brands of the different countries with a daily consumption of 20 cigarettes were taken (19). For the Federal Republic of Germany these 3 brands have a total share of market of more than 40 % (13). Since the most popular cigarette brands generally have a moderate nicotine delivery the values determined under standard smoking conditions can be considered to represent the TSNA intake by smokers. The favourable situation in Great Britain with respect to NNN can be attributed to a high proportion of Virginia tobaccos (14,6), which are preferably consumed in that country (27).

SUMMARY

For relative risk evaluation the tar delivery alone is not a sufficient parameter for the carcinogenic potential and the biological activity of cigarette smoke, since it does not reflect the level of the strong carcinogens NNN and NNK, which can be present in mainstream smoke in rather high concentrations. NNN and NNK should be determined and declared as an additional and adequate parameter. Furthermore for relative risk evaluation of low nicotine cigarettes the increased intake of smoke constituents with increasing inhalation volume has to be considered. A reduction of smokers' burden with the strong carcinogens NNN and NNK is possible if tobaccos with low levels of preformed TSNA are chosen for cigarette manufacturing. As discussed above the level of preformed TSNA in tobacco is correlated with the nitrate level of tobacco. Thus only tobaccos low in nitrate should be selected and the portions of nitrate rich Burley tobaccos and tobacco stems should be reduced. Since the TSNA intake of smokers is dependent on the total volume drawn through a cigarette during smoking and consequently on the nicotine delivery of the cigarettes, manufacturing cigarettes with low NNN/nicotine and NNK/nicotine ratios would result in a further exposure reduction.

REFERENCES

1. International Agency for Research on Cancer IARC Monographs on the Evaluation of the Carcinogenic Risk of Chemicals to Humans. Tobacco smoking. (1986) Vol 38, Lyon, IARC.
2. Dube, M. F. and Green, C.R. (1982) Methods of collection of smoke for analytical purposes. Recent Adv Tobacco Sci, 8, 42-102.
3. Hoffmann, D. and Hecht SS. (1985) Nicotine derived N-nitrosamines and tobacco related cancer: current status and future directions. Cancer Res, 45, 935-944.
4. Hecht, S.S., Chen, Ch.B., Ornaf, R.M., Jacobs, E., Adams, J.D. and Hoffmann, D. (1978) Reaction of nicotine and sodium nitrite: formation of nitrosamines and fragmentation of the pyrrolidine ring. J Org Chem, 43, 72-76.
5. Fischer, S. (1988). Untersuchungen zur Belastung von Rauchern mit tabakspezifischen Nitrosaminen und Moglichkeiten zur Expositionsverminderung. University of Heidelberg, FRG: Doctoral thesis.
6. Fischer, S., Spiegelhalder, B. and Preussmann, R. (1989) Preformed tobacco-specific nitrosamines in tobacco - role of nitrate and influence of tobacco type. 1989. Carcinogenesis, 10, 1511-1517.
7. Fischer, S., Spiegelhalder, B. and Preussmann, R. (1990) Tobacco-specific nitrosamines in European and USA cigarettes. Arch Geschwulstforsch, 60, 169-177.
8. Hecht, S.S. and Hoffmann, D. (1988) Tobacco-specific nitrosamines an important group of carcinogens in tobacco and tobacco smoke. Carcinogenesis, 9, 875-884.

9. LaVoie, E.J., Prokopczyk, G., Rigotty, J., Czech, A., Rivenson, A. and Adams, J.D. (1987) Tumorigenic activity of the tobacco-specific nitrosamines 4-(methylnitrosamino)-1-(3-pyridyl)-1-butanone (NNK), 4-(methylnitrosamino)-1-(3-pyridyl)-1-butanol (iso-NNAL) and N-nitrosonornicotine (NNN) on topical application to Sencar mice. 1987. Cancer Lett, 37, 277-283.
10. Verordnung uber Tabakerzeugnisse (Tabakverordnung) vom 20 December (1977) (BGBl. I S.2831) i.d.F. der AndV. vom 26.10.1982 (BGBl.I.S.1444).
11. Kommission der Europaischen Gemeinschaften Vorschlag uber eine Richtlinie des Rates zur Angleichung der Rechts- und Verwaltungsvorschriften der Mitlgliedsstaaten uber den hochstzulassigen Teergehalt von Zigaretten. (1988). Brussels, Belgium.
12. Klus, H. (1986) Low-tar cigarettes - possibilities and limitations. In: Zaridze D.G. and Peto, R. (eds) Tobacco: A major international health hazard. IARC Scientific Publication N. 74, Lyon France, pp 265-281.
13. Anonymus Die TabakZeitung, DTZ-Dokumentation N. 17, Mainz FRG. Mainzer Verlagsgesellschaft, (1988).
14. Fischer, S., Spiegelhalder, B. and Preussmann, R. (1989) Tobacco-specific nitrosamines in mainstream smoke of West germany cigarettes - tar alone is not a sufficient index for the carcinogenic potential of cigarette smoke. Carcinogenesis, 10, 169-173.
15. Ruhl, C., Amdas, J.D. and Hoffmann, D. (1980) Chemical studies on tobacco smoke. LXIV. Comparative assessment of volatile and tobacco-specific N-nitrosamines in the smoke of selected cigarettes from the USA, West Germany and France. J Anal Toxicol, 4, 255-259.
16. Chamberlain, W. J., Bates, J.C., Chortyk, O.T. and Stephenson, M.G. (1986) Studies on the reduction of nitrosamines in tobacco. Tobacco Sci, 81, 38-39.
17. Akehurst, B.C. (1981) Tobacco. London, New York: Longman.
18. Fischer, S., Spiegelhalder, B., Eisenbarth, J. and Preussmann, R. (1990) Investigations on the origin of tobacco-specific nitrosamines in mainstream smoke of cigarettes. Carcinogenesis, in press.
19. Anonymous How the brands ranked. (1987) World Tob, 100, 72-74.
20. Fischer, S., Spiegelhalder, B. and Preussmann, R. (1989) Influence of smoking parameters on the delivery of tobacco-specific nitrosamines in cigarette smoke - a contribution to relative risk evaluation. Carcinogenesis, 10, 1059-1066.
21. Herning, R. I., Jones, R.T., Bachman, J. and Mines, A.H. (1981). Puff volume increases when low-nicotine cigarettes are smoked. Brit Med J, 282, 187-189.
22. Puustinen, P., Olkkonen, H., Kolonen, S. and Tuomisto,

J. (1987) Microcomputer-aided measurement of puff parameters during smoking of low- and medium-tar cigarettes. Scand J Clin Lab Invest, 47, 655-660.

23. Russel, M. A. H. (1976) Low-tar medium-nicotine cigarettes: a new approach to safer smoking. Br Med J, 1, 1430-1433.

24. Woodman, G., Newman, S. P., Pavia, D. and Clarke, S. W. (1987) The separate effects of tar and nicotine on the smoking manoeuvre. Eur J Respir Dis, 70, 316-321.

25. Hoffmann, D., Dong, M. and Hecht, S. S. (1977) Origin in tobacco smoke of N'-nitrosonornicotine a tobacco-specific carcinogen: brief communication. J Natl Canc Inst, 58, 1841-1844.

26. Adams, J. D., Lee, S. J., Vinchkoski, N., Castonguay, A. and Hoffmann, D. (1983) On the formation of the tobacco-specific carcinogen 4-(methylnitrosamino)-1--(3-pyridyl)-1-butanone during smoking. Cancer Lett, 17, 339-346.

27. Borland, C. and Higenbottam, T. (1987) Nitric oxide yields of contemporary UK, US and French cigarettes. Int J Epidemiol, 16, 31-34.

10

MALIGNANT MELANOMA: AN EPIDEMIOLOGICAL PHENOMENON

F J Lejeune (a,b), **D Lienard** (a), **J Andre** (b,c) **M Joarlette** (a), **R Sacre** (b,d),
M Dramaix (e), **D Roseeuw** (f), **A Verhest** (b,g), **G Achten** (c)
(a)   L O C E, Institut Bordet, Brussels;
(b)   EORTC Malignant Melanoma Cooperative Group;
(c)   Service de Dermatologie, Hôpital Saint-Pierre, Brussels;
(d)   Service de Chirurgie, AZ-VUB, Brussels;
(e)   Ecole de Santé Publique, ULB, Brussels;
(f)   Service de Dermatologie, AZ-VUB, Brussels;
(g)   Service d'Anatomie Pathologique, Hôpital Erasme, Brussels

INTRODUCTION

Malignant melanoma is one of the few cancers still
increasing in incidence and mortality. The National Cancer
Institute figures show that its mortality rate increases by
1.8% per year; for the decade 1975-1984, mortality increased
by 23% in males and 10% in females. In the year 1983,
melanoma was the second cause of death from cancer in people
younger than 35 years.

In Europe, we are lacking overall figures but
Scandinavian and Scottish figures point to an increase of
both incidence and mortality during the past 20 years.

It is well known that basal cell carcinomas (the most
frequent skin cancers) as well as spindle cell carcinomas
result, late in life, from the cumulative effect of
ultraviolet (UV) exposure. More recently, the alarming
increase of malignant melanoma among white population in
Australia has permitted the discovery of the role of flash
exposure and, to a lesser degree, of cumulative UV as
aetiologic factors.

Epidemiological studies are therefore strongly needed
for assessing the role of UV light in melanomas occurring in
Europe.

UV EXPOSURE AND MELANOMA

The fraction of the solar radiation which contains UV-rays starts at 100 nanometers (nm), the border of X-rays and ends at 400 nm, the border of visible light. The biomedical literature used to divide UV into three types: UVC, UVB and UVA.

UVC (100 to 290 nm) are the most energetic. They used to be almost totally absorbed by the ozone layer of the atmosphere but, recently, it has been shown that the latter is being steadily destroyed and some holes have been detected (1-3). This finding is frightening as UVC are lethal, being able, for example, to destroy microorganisms very rapidly. Although UVC are mainly absorbed by the stratum corneum of the epidermis, they can induce severe DNA damage.

UVB (290 to 320 nm) are partly absorbed by the earth atmosphere (4,5). Between 6 and 10 am and 2 and 7 pm, there is almost no UVB radiation on the earth surface, whilst there is maximum radiation at solar midday. UVB penetrate into the human epidermis and reach the superficial dermis. The immediate action is well known: namely "sun burn" or actinic erythema. Solar minimum erythema is used as a reference standard for measuring UV radiation and antisolar protections, as it results from many complex factors. MED (Minimal Erythema Dose) corresponds to the quantity of UV capable of inducing a minimal erythema with clearcut borders.

UVA (320 to 400 nm) are almost unabsorbed by the atmosphere. For their poor capacity to induce erythema, they have been considered for a long time to be innocuous. They are currently produced artificially and intensively by solar UV lamps, well known as tanning cabinets. In contrast to UVC and UVB, UVA penetrate deeply into human skin: 30% reach the dermis and it has been shown that they can reach 2 mm in depth (6).

The natural UVA can reach the earths surface at any time and are capable of producing reactions which include photoactivation or photosensitization of molecules present in human skin. UVA radiation is in fact hazardous. One of the very few positive effects of UVA radiation is the stimulation of vitamin D synthesis. Melanogenesis, which is the melanin pigment synthesis, can be stimulated by UV, especially UVA, but there is growing evidence that skin tanning is not a sign of good health but rather a sign of human skin aggression followed by a protective reaction. When the sun is at its zenith, UVB irradiation represents only 8% of total UV energy against 92% for UVA (7). Therefore, UVA deserves special attention.

Many biological molecules are altered by activation in the presence of photosensitizing agents such as psoralens

and very often with oxygen. They are called photodynamic
reactions. Three major types have been recognized: type I or
free radical reactions; type II or energy transfer
reactions; and type III or chemical photosensitizing
reactions (8,9). Whilst oxygen is always involved in
reactions of types I (10,11) and II (12), it is unnecessary
for reaction III. Table I shows a short classification of
photosensitizing agents. The biochemical aspects (8) of
photosensitization are summarized in Table 2. The biological
and clinical aspects of UV-induced damages are summarized in
Table 3.
    The alarming effect of UV starts with sunburn erythema
and ends with skin aging due to elastotic neoformation. In
contrast, the great and insidious effect of overexposure to
UV is the induction of skin cancers including melanoma (15).

TABLE 1: Exogenous UVA photosensitizers.

A. Topical

    I Cosmetics, perfumes,   5-methoxypsoralen
      Soaps, creams   Dimethylan thralinate
      Sunscreens   7-methoxycoumarin
                                  Amyldimethylaminobenzoate

   II Pharmaceuticals
      Adverted   Psoralens, tars
      Inadverted   Polycyclic hydrocarbons
                                  (phenothiazines, e.g.
                                  chlorpromazine),
                                  Halogenated salicylamides

  III Plants
      Lime
      Celery   Furocoumarin
      Carrot   (including psoralens)
      Parsley

B. Systemic

I   Sulfonamides (antibacterial)
II   Thiazide diuretics
III   Sulfonylurea (antidiabetic)
IV   Phenothiazins (chlorpromazine sedative & anti-
      histaminic)
V   Tetracyclines (antibiotics)
VI   Coumarins (anticoagulants)
VII   Synthetized steroids (contraceptive)

Modified according to Epstein (13) and Kligman (14).

127

TABLE 2: Photosensitization : Biochemical aspects.

Global phenomenons

Substances	Effects
Carbohydrate	Little damaging
Unsaturated lipids	Allylic hydroperoxidation
Cholesterol	Hydroperoxidation
Proteins	Photooxydation

Particular phenomenons

Human serum + porphyrins	Inactivated hemolytic complement + C5 activation
Nucleic acids	DNA photooxydation Nucleic-proteins acids photoaddition
Phaeomelanins	Photoproducts (mutations)
Membranes	Permeability augmentation Lysis

TABLE 3: Photosensitization: Biological and clinical aspects.

Immediate reactions

Burning	Sunburn cells Inflammatory reaction
DNA alteration	Repairs Mutations

Melanocytes division
Keratinocytes alteration
Langerhans cells alteration or disappearance
Induction of suppressor T lymphocytes
Inhibition of T helper lymphocytes

Late reactions

Actinic aging
Solar elastosis
Benign keratoses
Telangectiasis

Actinic keratoses	atrophic hypertrophic Bowen

Spindle cell carcinoma
Basal cell carcinoma
Malignant melanoma

In a recent review of the literature on the relationship between UV and skin cancer, we have detected 7 groups of arguments which represent evidence for such an association (16). This review is summarized in Fig. 1.

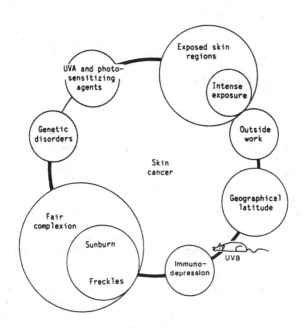

Figure 1.   Association of skin cancer with sun exposure.

The anatomic distribution of skin cancer shows a clearcut difference between carcinomas and melanomas. Whilst the first are located mainly in the head and neck region (basal cell carcinoma more than 70%, spindle cell carcinoma more than 40%), head and neck melanomas only represent 8.8% for females and 16.6 for males. Malignant melanomas of the lower limbs represent 53% of females and 29.3% of males whilst it is less than 1% for basal cell carcinomas and less than 6% for spindle cell carcinomas. Trunk melanomas occurred in 43% of males and 17.6% of females whilst it is less than 5% for carcinomas.

This discrepancy between carcinomas and melanomas is mainly due to the fact that carcinomas occur on chronically exposed skin, especially in farmers, sailors and railway employees, whilst melanomas seem to result from brief and intense exposure of cutaneous regions which are habitually covered by clothes (Table 4).

TABLE 4: Anatomical distribution of skin cancers (in %)

| Localisation | Cell carcinomas (a) | | | | Melanoma (b) | |
| | Basal | | Spindle | | | |
	M	F	M	F	M	
Head & neck	71.9	73.7	43.2	48.9	16.6	8.8
Upper limbs	1.9	1.6	1.5	0.5	10.6	20.6
Trunk	4.0	2.1	3.1	2.2	43.3	17.6
Lower limbs	0.7	0.5	5.0	3.3	29.3	53.0

(a) Silverstone and Seale (17)
(b) André et al (18)

The lower the latitude the higher the level of UV radiation. In Australia and USA, a direct correlation has been found between latitude and melanoma incidence. It has been recently claimed that it is of almost 40 for 100.000 inhabitants in south of USA and north of Australia. This is equal to the most common cancers.

The experimental evidence on mice is that UVB alone are able to produce DNA damage with strand breakage and sister chromatin exchange resulting in mutation and skin cancer (19-21). For UVA, it has been well documented that the application of photosensitizing agents such as psoralen, produce a very strong carcinogenic effect on nude mice. In the human, the evidence is still lacking but there are some reports suggesting the association between carcinomas and melanomas and the use of PUVA (psoralen and UVA) (10,22).

Immunodepression is a rather newly reported effect of UV. In the epiderm, the Langerhans cells, which are the macrophages of the skin, can be altered and strongly damaged. Blood cells irradiated when they flow in the skin can be altered by UVA: helper T lymphocytes and cytotoxic T lymphocytes can be depressed, suppressor T lymphocytes can be induced, presentation of antigen can be altered. Antibodies themselves can even be inactivated (23-29).

All human beings are not equal towards UVs. Table 5 shows the different phototypes and the UV dosis necessary to induce erythema.

Table 6 demonstrates the risk at developing a malignant melanoma according to the skin phototype. 407 melanoma cases were compared to 3062 doctors, nurses, workers, and hospital officers working in the Brussels ULB and VUB University Hospitals. Melanoma population has 1.6 fold more skin phototypes I and II than the control population (p<0.001). Although this was not a through case control study, odds ratio can be calculated. Table 6 demonstrates that the difference between phototypes I and III is the highest risk but it is still present between phototypes II and III. In contrast, there was no difference between phototypes I and IV which may suggest that melanomas occurring on phototype IV people are not a result of UV carcinogenesis.

TABLE 5: Cutaneous phototypes (a)

Type	Solar reaction	Minimum erythemal dosis (b)
	From 12 to 40 years	in microW/sec/cm^2
I	Always burns, never tans	3.74×10^5
II	Always burns, sometimes tans	6.26×10^5
III	Sometimes burns, always tans	9.35×10^5
IV	Never burns, always tans	1.47×10^6
V	Pigmented	
VI	Black	3.62×10^6

(a) Parrish et al (33)
(b) Urbach et al (34)

TABLE 6: Phototypes

Phototypes	Melanoma (407) %	Control (3062) %	Odds ratio		
I (198)	14.7	4.5	!	!	
II (1003)	37.8	27.7	!2.5	!6	!1
III (1910)	31.7	58.2	!	!	!
IV (358)	15.7	9.6			!

Therefore, phototypes represent a very useful marker for melanoma risk and it is worth diffusing this notion among not only the medical world but also the European populations.

An other marker at the risk of malignant melanoma development seems to be the number of naevi as reported independently by Armstrong (30) in Australia and Osterlind (31) in Denmark. Fig. 2 shows that the relative risk at developing melanoma increases according to the number of naevi. It is worth mentioning that it seems that the number of naevi is related to the sun exposure in the childhood

131

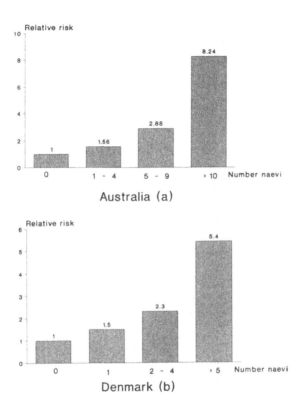

Australia (a)

Denmark (b)

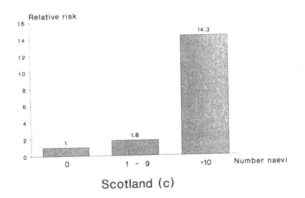

Scotland (c)

Figure 2: (a) English (ref 30), (b) Osterlind (ref 31), (c) Swerdlow (ref 32). Relative risk of melanoma according to the number of naevi on upper limb in Australia, Denmark and Scotland.

132

between birth and 10 years. Indeed, people born in Australia or in New-Zealand present a higher risk than immigrants who came after the age of 10 or 15 (Table 7).

The study of Swerdlow (32) in Scotland also points out the risk related to the number of naevi and also the inability to tan and develop freckles.

TABLE 7: Relative risk to develop melanoma
```
-----------------------------------------------------
                          0-9 years   > 10 years
Coming in Australia           1          0.38      Incidence
          New Zeeland          1          0.5       Mortality
-----------------------------------------------------
```

EARLY DIAGNOSIS

In malignant melanoma, the most significant criterion for prognosis is the primary tumour thickness as measured according to Breslow. In the Melanulb-Melavub study, it appears that females presented with thinner melanoma than males (Table 8) and that the thinner were the melanomas, the younger were the patients (Table 9). Such differences may be due to the different reporting behaviour between sexes and age. As a matter of fact, most melanomas were symptomatic: 83% of patients reported an increase of size and 65% a change in pigmentation.

TABLE 8: Breslow thickness

Sex	N	Mean Breslow	s.d.	p
Male	111	1.99	1.68	
Female	208	1.74	2.04	.02

Mann-Whitney

TABLE 9: Age & Breslow thickness

Breslow thickness (mm)	N	Mean age	s.d.	F	p
< .75	96	46.2	15.5		
.75-1.5	95	48.1	13.7		
1.51-3	78	48.6	15.2		
> 3	50	54.2	18.6	2.79	.032

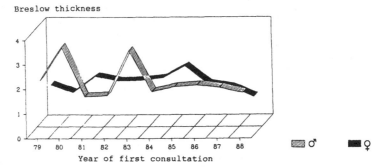

Figure 3: Breslow thickness evolution between 1979 and 1987.
Mean Breslow thickness by year of first consultation.

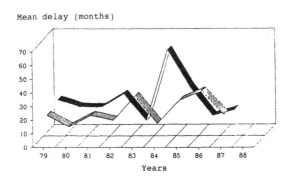

Figure 4a: First consultation delay. All delays.

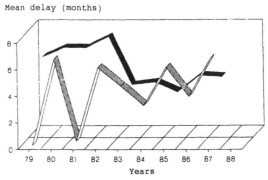

Figure 4b: First consultation delay. Delay $\leq$ 12 months.

We addressed the question as to whether information campaigns that we have organized in Belgium since 1983 would have had an impact on reporting delay. Fig. 3 shows that no significant difference in Breslow thickness was detected between 1979 and 1987. Moreover, a study on first consultation delay revealed no significant trend in the same period (Fig. 4a and 4b). In contrast, our data suggest that people with unfavourable phototypes reported quicker than people with better ability to tan (Table 10). Whether delay before diagnosis worsens prognosis is not fully demonstrated. In our series, there was a trend: the mean reporting delay was 24 months for melanomas less or equal to 3 mm thickness, 38 months for more than 3 mm.

TABLE 10: Consultation delay $\leq$ 12 months & phototypes

Phototype	N	Mean	s.d.	p
I	40	2.7	3.9	
II	93	5.1	4.6	
III	86	5.4	4.9	
IV	42	6.1	4.6	
Total	261	5.0	4.6	.002

Kruskall-Wallis

CONCLUSIONS

Such findings need to be confirmed on a pan-European basis.
The EORTC (European Organization for Research and Treatment of Cancer) Malignant Melanoma Cooperative Group will jointly implement with the SEARCH Programme of the IARC (International Agency for Research on Cancer) in Lyon, a prospective case-control study.
Besides exogenous factors, dysplastic naevi seem to represent an important risk factor either genetically linked or not. The EORTC Melanoma Group and SEARCH Programme will also initiate a prospective cohort study, based on 100.000 family members where about 10% histologically confirmed dysplastic naevi cases are anticipated.

REFERENCES

1. Jones, R.R. (1987). Ozone depletion and cancer risk. The Lancet, Aug. 22, 443-446.
2. Norman, C. (1981). Satellite data indicate ozone

depletion. Science, 213, 1088-1089.

3. Redman, J.C. (1987). Stratospheric ozone depletion. A proposed solution to the problem. Am J Dermopathol, 9, 457-458.

4. Cesarini, J.P., Robert, P. (1985). Rayons ultraviolets. In: "Dermopharmacologie clinique" (ed. Robert, P.) pp. 223-231, Paris, Maloine.

5. Pathak, M.A., Harber, L.C., Seiji, M. et al. (1974). "Sunlight and man" (eds. Pathak, M.A. et al), Tokyo, University of Tokyo Press.

6. Bruls, W.A.G., Slaper, H., Van der Leun, J.C., et al. (1984). Transmission of human epidermis and stratum corneum as a function of thickness in the ultraviolet and visible wavelength. Photochem Photobiol, 40, 485-494.

7. Cesarini, J.P. (1986). Le soleil et l'homme: physique et physiologie. Tribune médicale, 189, 13-18.

8. Spikes, J.D. (1983). Photosensitized reactions in mammals. In: "Experimental and clinical photo-immunology", Vol. 1, (eds. Daynes, R.A. and Spikes, J.D.) pp. 69-80, Boca Raton, CRC Press.

9. Willis, I. (1983). Ultraviolet light and skin cancer. In: "Experimental and clinical photoimmunology", Vol. II (eds. Daynes, R.A. and Krueger, G.) pp. 131-144, Boca Raton, CRC Press.

10. Stern, R.S. (1989). PUVA and the induction of skin cancer. Carcinog Compr Surv, 11, 85-101.

11. Baker-Blocker, A. (1980). Ultraviolet radiation and melanoma mortality in the United States. Environm Res, 23, 24-28.

12. Beitner, H., Ringborg, U., Wennersten, G. et al (1981). Further evidence for increased light sensitivity in patients with malignant melanoma. Br J Dermatol, 104, 289-294.

13. English, D.R., Heenan, P.J., D'Arcy, J. et al (1987). Melanoma in Western Australia in 1980-1981: incidence and characteristics of histological types. Pathology, 19, 383-392.

14. Kligman, A.M., Kaidbey, K.H. (1982). Human models for identification of photosensitizing chemicals. JNCI, 69, 269.

15. Young, L.F. (1981). Melanomas and sunlight. Med J Aust, 2, 258.

16. Lejeune, F.J., Joarlette, M. (1989). Soleil et cancer. Encyclopédie Médico-chirurgicale, 50035 A14-9, 1-10.

17. Silverstone, H., Searle, J.H.A. (1970). The epidemiology of skin cancer in Queensland. Br J Cancer, 24, 235-253.

18. André, J., Joarlette, M., Villar, J., Liénard, D., Verhest, A. et al (1989). Descriptive epidemiology of 415 cases of malignant melanomas observed in Brussels, Belgium in the eighties. Second International Conference

on Melanoma, Venice, Italy, Fondazione Giorgio Cini, October 16-19, 1989.

19. Urbach, F., Epstein, J.H., Forbes, P.D. (1974). Ultraviolet carcinogenesis: experimental, global, and genetic aspects. In:"Sunlight and man", (eds. Pathak, M.A. et al) pp.259-283, Tokyo, University of Tokyo Press.

20. Forbes, P.D. (1981). Photocarcinogenesis: an overview. J Invest Dermatol, 77, 139-143.

21. Van der Leun, J.C. (1984). UV-carcinogenesis. Photochem Photobiol, 39, 861-868.

22. Amblard, P., Beani, J.C., Reymond, J.L., Didier-Roberto, B. (1987). Photocarcinogenesis. Ann Dermatol Venereol, 114, 381-394.

23. Bergstresser, P.R., Streilein, J.W. (1983). Local effects of ultraviolet radiation on Langerhans cells and contact hypersensitivity. In: "Experimental and clinical photoimmunology", Vol. II (eds. Daynes, R.A. and Krueger, G.) pp. 37-49, Boca Raton, CRC Press.

24. Lynch, D.H., Gurish, M.F., Daynes, R.A. (1983). Modification of lymphocyte and macrophage functions in vitro following UVL exposure. In: "Experimental and clinical photoimmunology", Vol. II (eds. Daynes, R.A. and Krueger, G.) pp. 71-88, Boca Raton, CRC Press.

25. Green, M.I., Sy, M.S., Kripke, M. et al (1979). Impairment of antigen-presenting cell function by ultraviolet radiation. PNAS, 73, 6591.

26. Kraemer, K.H., Levis, W.R., Cason, J.C. et al (1981). Inhibition of mixed leukocyte culture reaction by 8-methoxypsoralen and long-wave-length ultraviolet radiation. J Invest Dermatol, 77, 235.

27. Lindhal-Kiessling, K., Safwenberg, J. (1971). Inability of UV-irradiated lymphocytes to stimulate allogeneic cells in mixed lymphocyte culture. Int Arch Allergy, 41, 670.

28. Moscicki, R., Morison, W., Bloch, K.J. et al (1981). Distribution of T cell subsets, identified by monoclonal antibodies in psoriasis treated with psoralen/ultra-violet-A radiation (PUVA). Clin Res, 29, 373A.

29. Sprangrude, G.J., Daynes, R.A. (1983). Oxygenated sterols as immunosuppressive agents. In: "Experimental and clinical photoimmunology", Vol. II (eds. Daynes, R.A. and Krueger, G.) pp. 89-102, Boca Raton, CRC Press.

30. Holman, C.J., Armstrong, B.K., Heenan, P.J. (1983). A theory of the etiology and pathogenesis of human cutaneous malignant melanoma. JNCI, 71, 651.

31. Osterlind, A., Tucker, M.A., Hou-Jensen, K., Stone, B.J., Engholm, G., Jensen, O.M. (1988). The Danish case-control study of cutaneous malignant melanoma. I. Importance of host factors. Int J Cancer, 42, 200.

32. Swerdlow, A.J., English, J., MacKie, R., O'Doherty, C.J., Hunter, J.A.A., Clark, J., Hole, D.J. (1986).

Benign melanocytic naevi as a risk factor for malignant melanoma. Brit Med J, 292, 1555-1559.

33. Parrish, J.A., White, H.A.D., Pathak, M.A. (1979). Photomedicine. In: "Dermatology in general medicine. Textbook and atlas" (eds. Fitzpatrick, T.B. et al) pp. 942-994, New York, McGraw-Hill Book Company.

34. Urbach, F. (1981). Skin cancer in man. a) Geographical and racial variations. In: "Biology of skin cancer (excluding melanoma)" A series of Workshops on the Biology of Human Cancer, report n.15. UICC Technical Report Series, Vol. 63 (eds. Laerum, O.D. et al) pp. 58-66 and 80-86, Geneva, UICC.

11
HEALTHY EATING AND PUBLIC EDUCATION

J V Wheelock
Food Policy Research Unit, Department of Biomedical Sciences,
University of Bradford, Bradford, West Yorkshire BD7 1DP, United Kingdom

Studies on how food consumption patterns evolve based on data from many different countries show that there is a characteristic series of change in diet and in the factors which influence the choice of food (1).

In an agrarian society, most of the food is produced by those who consume it. The type of food available is therefore largely determined by what can be grown in the locality. As industrialisation progresses and people leave the land to work in the urban areas, many of the links between production and consumption are broken. Food has to be purchased by a growing proportion of the population and so economic factors - prices and incomes - take over as the main influence determining food choice. Improvements in living standards are usually associated with a steady increase in the proportion of animal products in the diet. At the same time, the proportion of income spent on food declines. In Britain today it is about 18% (including expenditure on food consumed outside the home) (2).

During the last 30 years, one of the major features of the British diet has been a growth in the consumption of convenience foods and convenience meals. In effect, the food processing industries have taken over much of food preparation that was previously done in the home. Undoubtedly, this has occurred because of the growth of number of married women now in employment.

More recently, it has become evident that the amount of foods of animal origin in the diet of many countries has reached a peak and there are indications that the demand for milk, meat, eggs and their products may actually be falling. Furthermore, there is considerable variation between individuals in what they actually eat. This is because the modern supermarkets are, in general, very spacious so that they can have as many as 18,000 different food products compared with as few as 400 products in the early supermarkets about thirty years ago. As a result, consumers can usually select those food products which most closely meet their own personal requirements.

In addition, supermarkets are continually monitoring the changes in consumer attitudes, and if they identify an unsatisfied demand, they are quite likely to seek out the requisite new products. For consumers, this means that they can now choose from a very wide range. It is easy to try out new products. Because the total amount of food consumed is relatively static, any increase in demand for one product must mean there is a concomitant fall in sales of some other product. Hence the modern food markets are very volatile. At the same time, price has become much less important as a factor influencing food choice. Consumers are prepared to pay a premium for quality or, perhaps more accurately, for what they believe is quality. Many different characteristics and opinions contribute to an individual's perception of quality so there can be marked variations between people in their view of quality. Nevertheless, it is evident that health aspects are an important dimension of quality and increasingly are having an impact on food choice.

The big problem for consumers is that they are being subjected to a variety of different messages which relate to diet and health. Not surprisingly, they find it extremely difficult to distinguish between advice which is based on a balanced objective interpretation of the scientific evidence and that which is not.

In order to consider the role of public education in people's views of healthy eating, it is necessary to consider some of the important types of information that help to shape an individual's knowledge of diet and health. Although there is considerable interaction and overlap between the different sources, it is appropriate to deal with this information under the following headings:

* The Food Industry
* The Media
* The Government

THE FOOD INDUSTRY

Nowadays the public is provided with much information on food and nutrition by the food industry. This can be in the form of packaging, advertising, leaflet and booklets. Some of these relate to specific commodities and are prepared by organisations which represent a sector of the industry. Others are confined to one company and its own products. In recent years, retailers have started producing booklets which do not necessarily focus on individual products or product ranges but are more likely to consider issues that will be of interest to their customers.

Packaging

Packages are usually designed to make them as attractive as possible, although there are legal requirements which specify certain information that must be given.
   Nevertheless, there is still scope for much more material to be incorporated especially in large products. With the growing interest in diet and health, it is now very common for certain characteristics of the food to be featured on the label, with the objective of influencing the shopper to buy the product. This may take the form of concise phrases such as:

> "A good source of calcium"
> "Low fat"
> "High in natural fibre"
> "No added salt"
> "No added sugar"
> "Approved by the Vegetarian Society"
> "No artificial colours or preservatives".

However, a number of products now provide quite detailed information on health related aspects. Recently, companies have been focusing on heart disease with particular reference to soluble fibre in oats (Boxes 1 and 2). Organically-grown products are considered to be environmentally-friendly and healthy. In Britain, there is a growing demand for such products (Box 3).

BOX 1

HOW OATS AND OAT BRAN HELP REDUCE CHOLESTEROL

   Oats and oat bran contain a very special kind of fibre - soluble fibre.
   Research has shown that foods rich in soluble fibre can - when added to a low fat, low cholesterol diet - reduce blood cholesterol by significantly greater amounts than would have been achieved by the diet alone.

   SOLUBLE FIBRE

   Soluble fibre isn't the same kind of fibre that acts as roughage and aids digestion. Soluble fibre is found in relatively few foods and only in small quantities.
   This is what makes oats and oat bran so important - because oats and, in particular, oat bran are among the best food sources of soluble fibre.

                                        Quaker Oats

BOX 2

HERE'S A GREAT NEW CEREAL

OAT BRAN FLAKES

A healthy heart is the key to a healthy body and the
key to a healthy heart is : <u>Exercise</u> and <u>a balanced diet</u> to
help maintain a health weight and keep the heart in good
order.

Here's some good news! Inside this packet is a great
new cereal - COMMON SENSE <u>OAT BRAN FLAKES</u> - that can help to
keep your heart in better shape.

Oat bran is a valuable source of soluble fibre, and
recent studies confirm that a regular intake of soluble
fibre as part of a fat modified diet can contribute towards
a reduction in blood cholesterol levels, and thus help to
prevent heart problems. Do you want to know more ? Well
here are the answers to a few questions ....

Kellogs Oat Bran Flakes

BOX 3

ORGANIC GRADE
Flavour by nature

Organic farming is a system which relies on good
husbandy and careful crop rotation by the farmer to maintain
the fertility and natural structure of the soil.

This is achieved by using natural organic fertilisers,
normally produced from within the farm, which improve and
enrich the soil, rather than synthetic fertilisers. No
chemical pesticides and herbicides which may damage the
environment are allowed.

All organic farms are monitored carefully by
independent inspectors and all crops certified to ensure
that they have been produced to organic standards.

Jordans Organic Multigram Puffed Cereals bring you the
flavour and goodness of three different cereals - wheat, rye
and rice. All of these grains derive their nutrients solely
from the combination of good healthy soil and the farmer
working in harmony with nature.

The whole grain cereals are simply puffed in an oven to
give them delightfully crisp texture and great taste.
Nothing else is added so you can be sure that Jordans
Organic Multigrain Puffed Cereals are pure in quality,
totally natural and good to eat.

PRODUCT OF AN ENVIRONMENTALLY SOUND FARMING SYSTEM

Jordans Organic Grade Puffed Cereals

142

It is also very common to have information on the nutritional composition of the product. In the UK, the Ministry of Agriculture, Fisheries and Food has prepared guidelines on how nutrition information should be presented but there are still many companies which prefer to use a different format to display the data.

Within the EC, there is at present no general EC-wide legislation on nutrition labelling and adoption ranges from rare, eg, Greece, to almost all packaged goods as in Denmark and Holland. The Commission published proposals on nutrition labelling in 1989 which:

a) Set out provisions enabling the EC (at some later date) to require nutrition labels to be provided; and

b) Set out rules for the presentation of nutrition labels when given voluntarily by manufacturers.

Despite the guidelines, there is still a wide variation in the way the nutrition information is presented (Tables 1 and 2). Hence it is very difficult for consumers to make comparisons between different products. For example, many dairy products do not give information on the types of fat present so that it is impossible to determine how much saturated fat is present.

TABLE 1: Fresh Pasteurised Milk

NUTRITION INFORMATION

TYPICAL VALUES PER 100 ML

Energy	280 kJ/67 kcal
Protein	3.4 g
Carbohydrate	4.8 g
Fat	3.9 g
Calcium	120 mg

                    Associated Fresh foods

A recent survey conducted by Alison Findlay in Bradford has established that there is much dissactifaction with the nutrition information and the way it is presented.

In the UK, a high proportion of the food is in the form of 'own label' - ie, specially produced by manufacturers for the retailers, in accordance with specifications laid down by the retailers. This includes the packaging and labelling. Tesco have recently altered their format (see Table 3) so that it now conforms to the official guidelines.

TABLE 2: Fresh Milk

```
-------------------------------------------
            NUTRITIONAL VALUES
        PER AVERAGE 100 ml SERVING

    Energy                  65 kcal/280 kJ
    Protein                    3.3 g
    Carbohydrate               4.7 g
    Total fat                  3.9 g
-------------------------------------------
              VITAMINS % OF
        RECOMMENDED DAILY AMOUNT
```

A	5%	Niacin	5%
Thiamin (B$_1$)	3%	B$_{12}$	15%
Riboflavin (B$_2$)	12%	calcium	25%

Dale Farm

Booklets and leaflets

In the UK, the National Dairy Council has produced a series of booklets. These include : "Off to a Fresh Start with Food and Fitness" which gives general advice on fitness and lifestyle. It then goes on to present some guidelines on healthy eating, pointing out that milk and milk products are valuable as a source of energy and important nutrients. Some examples of meals containing milk and dairy products are given which meet the official recommendations. Other booklets explain how it is possible to reduce total fat consumption by incorporating skim and semi-skimmed milk in the diet and the importance of milk in the diet as a source of calcium.

There is also a Nutritional Consultative Panel - "an independent group of nutrition experts which advises the dairy industry". This Panel produces Briefing Papers which are distributed to health professionals and other interested people. A recent issue on "Cholesterol in the Diet and Blood" "aims to describe what cholesterol is, why it is important in the body ...".

While much of the information is interesting and accurate, it simply ignores virtually all of the current evidence which leads to the conclusion that a high serum cholesterol level is a risk factor for coronary heart disease. For example, it states that "It is difficult to define an optimum concentration of cholesterol in the blood

TABLE 3: Tesco half fat fresh milk

NUTRITION
Tesco Semi-Skimmed Milk contains less than half the fat of whole milk while still containing the same quantity of protein, B vitamins and calcium. One pint provides the recommended daily amount of calcium.

Average composition	Per 568 ml (1 pint) serving	Per 100 ml (3.1/2 fl oz)
ENERGY	1130 kJ/270kcal	119 kJ/48 kcal
Fat	9.7 g	1.7 g
of which Saturates	6.2 g	1.1 g
Polyunsaturates	0.6 g	0.1 g
Protein	19.3 g	3.4 g
Carbohydrate	27.8 g	4.9 g

MINERALS/VITAMINS	% recommended daily amount	
Thiamin (Vitamin B_1)	19%	0.04 g
Riboflavine (Vitamin B_2)	71%	0.2 mg
Niacin	28%	0.9 mg
Vitamine B_{12}	114%	0.4 ug
Calcium	136%	120.0 mg

Tesco

... The range of blood cholesterol concentrations is much broader (than glucose) and the effects of straying much above or below "the normal range" are not readily apparent in the short term. Different communities may have widely different distributions of blood and this may depend on a combination of interacting factors including genetics, diet, personality, exercise patterns, and other aspects of lifestyle. In the UK, the average plasma cholesterol concentration is about 6 millimoles per litre of blood."
     There is no mention of the fact that the UK has one of the highest rates of CHD in the world and that countries with an average plasma cholesterol level of 4.5 millimoles per litre of blood or less do not have a high incidence of heart disease. There is no mention of the fact that there is almost unanimous agreement amongst the experts that it is highly desirable for individuals to reduce their blood cholesterol below 5.2 millimoles per litre of blood.

According to a United States Expert Panel (3): "Serum total cholesterol should be measured in all adults 20 years of age and over at least once every 5 years ...". "Levels below 5.2 millimoles/litre are classified as "desirable blood cholesterol", those 5.2 to 6.2 millimoles/litre as "borderline - high blood cholesterol" and those 6.2 millimoles/litre and above "high blood cholesterol".

This is because the risk of coronary heart disease rises progressively with cholesterol level, especially above 5.2 millimoles/litre. In fact, the Americans are so concerned that they have launched a massive National Cholesterol Education Program which is designed to reduce the incidence of coronary heart disease by encouraging individuals to have their blood cholesterol measured. If it is higher than the desirable level then changes in diet are recommended to help lower the cholesterol value.

The Briefing Paper also casts doubt on the desirability of lowering blood cholesterol by pointing out that : "a very low blood cholesterol has been associated with an increased risk of cancer". In fact, a major epidemiological study has examined mortality rates and biochemical characteristics of populations in 65 rural Chinese Counties (4). Even though plasma cholesterol was very low - in one group it was < 3.1 millimoles/litre - there was no evidence that those particularly low plasma cholesterol concentrations had high cancer rates. In fact, the authors conclude that cholesterol concentrations much lower than in Britain are not associated with any gross increase in cancer - indeed, if anything, the opposite trend was indicated (5).

The Federation of Bakers published a booklet entitled "Facts about Bread", which gives information about the different types of bread, the importance of fibre in the diet and the baking industry. It quotes official reports which point out that: "Bread contains protein, carbohydrate, calcium, iron and the B vitamins thiamin, niacin and a little riboflavine" and "Bread is a major source of fibre in the diet and provides more than a quarter of our daily intake".

The British Trout Information Bureau publish "Trim with Trout: For Your Health's Sake". The opening sentence is: "Trout forms the perfect basis for a healthy diet when combined with high fibre vegetables and fruit, and the energy-giving carbohydrates found in rice, wholemeal bread, potatoes and pasta."

Crosse & Blackwell have a leaflet "Healthy Balance" to provide information about the range of products which includes Baked Beans, Higher Fibre Spaghetti and Baked Beans with Low Fat Pork Sausages. Most of the leaflet is devoted to information on nutrition, nutrients and healthy eating.

"Living with Lo-Salt" deal specifically with the single product Lo-Salt. It explains why we should reduce sodium intake and how Lo-Salt can help achieve this by using it to replace ordinary table salt.

The Flora Project for Heart Disease Prevention is supported by Van den Berghs & Jurgens, the manufacturers of Flora margarine. One of their packs contains a series of leaflets which focus on the prevention of heart disease, as follows:

1. Exercise and Fitness
2. Blood pressure
3. Food Choices
4. Stress
5. Weight

Interestingly, none of these leaflets make any overt reference to Flora range of products.

Although most of the material described here is directed at the general public, companies also produce material specifically for health professionals.

It is well-known that manufacturers of infant formulae donate supplies to midwives and nurses - no doubt they find this a very effective way to promote their products.

Similarly, food manufacturers direct material at dieticians and teachers. However, studies conducted in Bradford by Nicholas HOWCROFT indicate that much of the material sent to schools is just not used by the teachers. Some teachers are suspicious that anything from the industry will lack objectivity and the prime reason is to advertise a company's product.

Others find that the packs of information do not fit into the curriculum and so it is not easy to incorporate them into a teaching programme.

One example which is likely to be effective is a teaching pack entitled Heinz Nutrition Workshop. The pack has been prepared in collaboration with Sheila TURNER and colleagues from the London Institute of Education. The stated aims are to help children to become aware of the huge range of foods avalaible; understand that they have choice about what they eat; appreciate the factors which influence their selection of food; and ultimately make informed choices about what they eat in full understanding of the relationship between diet and health. The material is free of any commercial bias and is aimed at schoolchildren between the ages of five and twelve.

At the retail end of the food chain, there have been many initiatives. In the United States, Giant Food Inc, which operates in the Maryland/Washington area, have pioneered the provision of high quality information for their customers. For example in 1982, they launched a booklet entitled "Calling a Halt to Salt" which explained why many people need to reduce their salt intake. It then went on to give the major sources of salt in the diet and to suggest what steps might be taken to lower salt consumption.

Finally, there is a detailed bibliography. Throughout the 1980s, Giant Food has taken a very positive approach towards its customers by making available information on a wide variety of issues.

In Britain, Tesco Stores launched a Healthy Eating Programme at the beginning of 1985. As part of this programme, a series of leaflets under the general heading - 'A Tesco Guide to Healthy Eating' on topics such as salt, protein, fibre, fat and sugar were prepared for free distribution in their stores.

Sainsbury's also have a series of leaflets dealing with a variety of topics such as :
"Your Food and Your Health"
"Keep Food at its Best"
"Understanding Food Labels"
"Sensible Drinking"

In Ireland, Superquin and the Irish Heart Foundation combined to produce a leaflet "Good Eating Does Your Heart Good" which gave advice on healthy eating.

Advertising

A high proportion of a food company's budget can be spent on marketing support. For example in the UK :
- Fanta has a 4 million Sterling pounds television in 1990.
- Birds Eye is spending 8 million Sterling pounds on its Healthy Options range of products. This will be used for press advertising, nation-wide poster campaign, which is the most that has ever been spent on a food launch in the UK.
- In 1989, Van den Bergs and Jurgens committed 5 million Sterling pounds to support the Flora brand.
- Coca Cola & Schweppes Beverages will spend 80 million Sterling pounds on marketing support for its brands, of which 30 million Sterling pounds will be spent on Coca-Cola during 1990.

Advertising can include posters, promotions such as sporting events, eg, the London Marathon has been sponsored by Mars, advertisements in shops, magazines, newspapers, radio and television. Obviously, companies believe that it is important to keep their products in the public eye. Furthermore, there can be very high costs involved in launching a new product, even though it has been shown that the success rate is very low. This demonstrates that advertising alone is no guarantee of success in the market place, although at least one product, the Walls Cornetto, had to be launched three times before it achieved a viable level of sales.

With the expanding use of scanning at supermarket check-outs, the scope for monitoring the effectiveness of advertising has been increased significantly. This is because it is now possible to follow the impact of any promotion very precisely and different approaches can be tested in different areas and the results compared.

THE MEDIA - Newspapers, magazines, books, radio and television

While most of the media acts as a vehicle for food marketing, the programmes and articles have also a very powerful influence on the readers, listeners and viewers. When an issue is suddenly the subject of media attention, such as salmonella in eggs, or listeria in paté, the combined effect can have a marked depression on the sales of food. In the UK, the two issues above resulted in a sharp fall in demand for eggs and for paté. Four years ago, there was a scare in Sweden about campylobacter in chickens, which caused a 40% decline in demand for chicken meat. In 1984, a programme about heart disease in Britain emphasised the desirability of reducing consumption of saturated fat, and as a result, there was a marked increase in demand for semi-skimmed (low-fat) milk as consumers switched away from full-fat milk.

The major problem with the media is that the reliability of information is extremely variable, and few people have the ability to be critical because they simply lack the specialised expertise. To scientists familiar with the system of peer review for the academic literature, the standard of quality control is very poor.

In my view, the main reasons for this are as follows:
- Most journalists do not have expertise possessed by scientists. Many writers on food topics may be responsible for the section dealing with cookery and may well be expected to produce articles dealing with quite complex aspects of nutrition. It is noteworthy that in Britain, writers on food topics do not usually have the degree of competence approaching those who would write on finance.
- Most articles have to be produced within a very limited time-scale. This applies especially to new items. If a story first emerges at 2 o'clock in the afternoon that is likely to be of great interest. For example, if high levels of aflatoxin in nuts are discovered and substantial quantities have been purchased and possibly consumed, then all the news programmes will expect to include an in-depth item within the next few hours - particularly in the main early evening news. People will want to know what are the risks to their health if they have eaten any of the nuts, what they should do if they are at risk, and any other advice that may be relevant. The journalist(s) allocated to the story will have to work very quickly indeed. There

simply will not be the time to do detailed research by finding and reading the fundamental scientific papers.

- Journalists are critically dependent on their existing contacts or whoever they can find <u>in the time available</u>. Inevitably, they will gravitate towards those who are well-known, who are articulate and who are available. These are not necessarily scientists who are reliable and accurate. In fact, many scientists are reluctant to make comments to the media because they are worried that their remarks may be misinterpreted. The position is exacerbated because journalists often want straight "YES/NO" answers, when the most accurate answers are "YES, BUT ...", "MAYBE ..." or "WE DO NOT KNOW". In fact, more often than not, scientists simply do not know enough to be able to give a definitive answer.

- If there is a possibility of a hazard to human health then consumers, politicians and journalists will expect and demand answer because it may be necessary to introduce control measures. An excellent example is provided by the current worries about bovine spongiform encephalopathy (BSE). We really know very little about the possibility that the agent will cross the trans-species boundary and infect humans, but still decisions have to be taken in the need for control measures. Under these circumstances, it is not in the least surprising that much of the coverage in the media is inaccurate and distorted.

- Journalists and their editors are primarily interested in making an impact which will sell their newspapers and magazines or encourage people to watch their programme. Sales, viewing and listening figures determine the charges for advertising (where this applies). Stories about foods that are dangerous tend to stimulate more interest than those which emphasise the safety of food. Complex issues are often simplified so that a distorted picture is presented. Frequently, food or food ingredients are described as being "carcinogenic" or "causes cancer in laboratory animals", yet it is very rare for any attempt to be made to explain what the actual risks may be for the human population. Such stories can be presented as though they are either a serious hazard or a negligible one.

- Journalists are usually free to purvey their own prejudices. In Britain, last September, there were several stories about the hazards that might be caused by polyunsaturated fatty acids. These were based on a misinterpretation of results from an experiment in Cambridge. Subsequently, the investigator disassociated himself from the journalist's conclusions.

150

GOVERNMENT

Agencies

The information from these sources tends to be relatively limited and so the impact, at least in the UK, is small when compared with that of the food industry and the media.

In England and Wales, the Health Education Authority provides information and organises campaigns promoting a healthy lifestyle. Some of these resources is directed towards the general public using the same methods and outlets as the food industries but on a very much smaller scale. Information is also provided for health and education professions.

At local and regional levels, health authorities have health promotion units which work within their own area of jurisdiction. The Yorkshire Regional Health Authority has prepared a booklet entitled "Coronary Heart Disease: Yorkshire's Biggest Killer" which is part of a prevention programme "Heartbeat Yorkshire" designed to reduce the incidence of heart disease.

Local authorities in Britain sometimes promote healthy eating. Tameside Metropolitan Borough in the Manchester area has a school catering service which is very positive in its promotion of healthy eating, although it has to be recognised that this is something of an exception.

Government sometimes produce materials which is aimed at the general public. For example, in Britain, a booklet entitled "Food Safety - A guide from H M Government" has recently been produced and given wide distribution.

In the United States, the Food Safety Inspection Service of the Department of Agriculture issues a series of publications, such as "The Safe Food Book : Your Kitchen Guide".

Leaflets include: "Know your Molds" - "Keeping Meat and Poultry Safe in Foul Weather".

The National Institutes of health have produced a leaflet dealing with cancer, entitled: "Diet, Nutrition and Cancer Prevention: The Good News".

Schools

Research in Bradford by Nicolas HOWCROFT has shown that in Britain all pupils in the Third Form (13-year old) do have some lessons in nutrition and healthy eating. Subsequently, only those pupils who choose to study Home Economics or Biology will receive any instruction in nutrition. In his studies, Nicolas HOWCROFT found that all the teachers he interviewed were very concerned that many children do not have a good background in nutrition, food safety and healthy eating. As a consequence, many of them are, effectively, left to learn for themselves. This means that they have to guage for themselves the bias in advertising, develop skills in safe food handling, as well as evolving the ability to construct a healthy diet.

The teachers were also very worried about the impact of the school tuck shop and the school meals service which frequently undermined their efforts to promote healthy eating. In tuck shops, the most commonly stocked items are crisps, biscuits and confectionery. The prime reasons is that these products have a high profit margin and in most schools, the object of the tuck shop is to raise extra income for school activities, such as maintenance of the school minibus.

School meal services are under pressure to give the pupils what they want, and so there is a tendency to provide meals with items such as chips, burgers and sausages. Some caterers complain that when they provide healthy meals they are expensive and that the pupils do not find them attractive. However, when a positive, imaginative approach is taken as in Tameside, this can be very successful.

This research also found that most teachers were fairly sceptical about the information from food manufacturing companies. By contrast, most of them were favourably impressed by the material available from the major retailers, mainly because it was easily understandable by pupils and it did not promote specific products.

DISCUSSION

The big problem for consumers is that they are being sujected to a variety of different messages which relate to diet and health. Not surprisingly, they find it extremely difficult to distinguish between advice which is based on a balanced objective interpretation of the scientific evidence and that which is not.

Food companies and food marketing organisations are responsible for an enormous amount of information in the public domain. There are food labels, advertisements in newspapers, magazines, radio and television; leaflets and booklets which are directed towards the public and the professions. In addition, food companies often have their own public relations departments and employ public relations agencies to send out a steady stream of press releases and to brief journalists. Much of the material is very well presented and, undoubtedly, finds its way into the non-advertising sectors.

From the perspective of those wishing to promote healthy eating, much of the marketing is not particularly helpful. In fact, it can be criticised quite heavily because as a whole, the impact of the key recommendations are diluted by messages which are peripheral or distorted.

For example, in Britain during the last few years, there has been interest in and concern about food additives. Products are being promoted as having "no artificial additives" or "natural colours" or "no preservatives". Additives are now subject to tight legislation control and, to the best of our knowledge, do not present any real hazards to the population as a whole. It is much more likely to be the reverse. Preservatives suppress the growth of pathogenic bacteria. Anti-oxidants can act as free radical traps in the body and prevent the deterioration of unsaturated fatty acids. As a general rule, natural colours have not been subjected to the same degree of testing as artificial colours and, therefore, could pose a greater risk.

Many foods are being promoted as "natural", because this is a feature consumers find attractive. They are usually perceived as wholesome and nutritious. Organically-grown foods are in big demand, despite the fact that some of them may be contaminated with pathogenic organisms such as listeria. Furthermore, some strains of plants which have been developed because of their pest resistance have actually been too dangerous to put on the market because of the high content of natural toxins present, presumably to act against predators. According to Bruce AMES (6) we should be much more concerned about the naturally-occurring pesticides present in fruits and vegetables than about the residues of pesticides applied by farmers and growers.

What is actually happening is that those marketing foods will make use of any characteristics that will help to portray an image of health. As a consequence, a food such as butter can be promoted as natural and free of additives, while there is no mention of the fact that there is a very high content of saturated fat.

It is important to recognise that there is a fundamental difference between the manufacturers and the retailers. Manufacturers produce a limited range of foods. They usually have a very heavy investment in specialist employees, technological expertise and dedicated plant. Hence they are effectively "locked in" to their existing range. Any major change in what is produced will be expensive in terms of time, effort and resources.

By contrast, the retailers are in a very different position. While they obviously want to sell food products, a key element in their marketing is to attract shoppers into their stores and to persuade them to keep coming back. Quality of service, range of products, attractiveness of stores all contribute to their success with customers. Most of the foods are obtained from suppliers who are under contract to the retailer. This means that it is very easy to vary the product range. If it is apparent that a product is not selling well, the relevant buyer simply terminates the contract. Similarly, arrangements can be made with suppliers for the provision of new or different products.

From the perspective of the retailers, there is not the same imperative to support any particular product. If they decide that they should provide information to consumers on dietary guidelines or food safety, it is highly probable that they will be balanced and objectivee in their selection and presentation of material. It is in their interests to do so, since this creates an image of caring and responsibility that ultimately will be good for business.

As explained earlier, the quality information provided in books, magazines, newspapers, radio and television is very variable and also has a powerful influence on consumers. As with the information put out by the food companies, the public is faced with the same difficulties in that few have the capability of evaluating what is presented to them.

The position would be alleviated if the population generally was well-informed about the issues and, therefore, possessed the skills to select the good from the bad. Unfortunately, this is not the case. The amount of information and education provided by government and public bodies is very limited, especially when compared to the other two sources. In Britain, the nutrition budget of the Health Education Authority is probably less than the marketing budget for one of the well-known brands of food.

Within the National Health Service, the amount of money spent on health promotion is very small when compared with what is spent on curative medicine. Promoting haelthy eating does not have the same appeal or urgency as spending money on expensive intensive care units which are equipped with all the latest technology. The fact that the impact of a good quality prevention programme would be infinitely greater in terms of reducing the incidence of disease seems to be irrelevant.

Although there are initiatives to encourage general practitioners to place more emphasis on prevention, including healthy eating, there is still a major problem because doctors have little training in nutrition and many of them are poorly informed about the basic dietary recommendations.

In schools, the prognosis is pessimistic. Healthy eating does not have a high priority in the curriculum. Where individuals teachers are being positive and enthusiastic, they often find that their efforts are undermined by the existence of a school tuck shop and a school meal service which is more concerned with economics than with nutrition.

THE WAY AHEAD

Although the picture, based largely on the experience in Britain, is not very encouraging, this is certainly not universal. If we take coronary heart disease as a model, good progress has been made in several countries, including Finland and Norway. In both of these, there has been considerable emphasis on the need for making changes to the diet. Clearly, there is scope for analysing and evaluating what has been achieved in these countries to determine what lessons can be learned which can be applied more widely.

In my view, there are three elements that need attention:

1. The results of scientific investigations must be evaluated and the implications for dietary recommendations worked out. Reports prepared by government bodies and scientific associations must be widely available so that they can act as a source of reference for government, industry and health professions.

2. The scientists doing the work must be prepared to take a much more active part in the public debate to ensure that there is a significant input which is balanced and objective. However, scientists must also recognise that they have a responsibility to be very careful in the statement they make in public. Scientists who make media contributions based on data which has not been subject to peer review can and do add to the state of public confusion.

3. Governments need to be pro-active. However, this is very dependent on the scientists agreeing on the strategies that should be adopted and being prepared to press the case for action in the official circles.

REFERENCES

1. Wheelock, J. V., Frank, J.D., Freckleton, A. and Hanson, L. (1987). Food consumption patterns and nutritional labelling in selected developed countries. Volume 1 FAST Occasional Paper N.130. Directorate-General for Science, Research and Development, Brussels: Commission of the European Communities.
2. Ministry of Agriculture, Ficheries and Food. (1989) Household food consumption and expenditure 1987 Annual Report of the National Food Survey Committee, London: HMSO.
3. Report of the Expert Pannel on Detection, Evaluation and Treatment of High Blood Cholesterol in Adults (1989). U.S. Department of Health and Human Services, Public Health Service, National Institute of Health, NIH Publication N. 89-2925, Washington DC.
4. Chen, J., Campbell, T.C., Li, J., Peto, R. (1989). Diet,

lifestyle and mortality in China. A study of characteristics of 65 Chinese Counties, Oxford University Press.

5. Peto, R., Boreham, J., Chen, J., Li, J., Campbell, T.C. and Brun, T. (1989). Plasma cholesterol, coronary heart disease, and cancer. Brit. Med. J., 298, 1249.

6. Ames, B.N., Magaw, R. and Gold, L.S. (1987). Ranking possible carcinogenic hazards, Science, 236, 271.

12

CANCER PRIMARY PREVENTION: A GAP BETWEEN KNOWLEDGE AND INTERVENTION

Attilio Giacosa
National Institute for Cancer Research, Genoa, Italy

Epidemiological observation of cancer prevalence in various geographic areas and of its relationship with life style as well as with multiple additional parameters helped to outline risk factors for cancer development. Moreover, studies of migrants and studies on anatomopathological patterns of cancer and precancerous lesions have been very helpful to define the multistep progression from normal tissue to cancer. The epidemiological approach to anatomopathology and growing evidences about biological markers of precancerous conditions has brought new knowledge on this matter.

Doll and Peto on the basis of the published evidences defined a well known table in which tobacco accounts for 30% of the whole cancer risk and diet for 35% of all cancers, but ranging from 10 to 70% according to different tumour sites.

The degree of uncertainty is still high for diet because in this field much of the information is still missing, while this is not the case for tobacco.

The choice of a primary or secondary preventive intervention should not be made on the basis of chance, but according to the biological and morphological features of the carcinogenetic process.

Obviously it will be impossible to formulate an effective primary prevention approach when the genetic involvement is high. Other conditions, such as breast and endometrial cancers, need secondary prevention because risk factors are not yet completely defined or cannot be easily removed (age at menarche, number of children, age at first birth, etc.).

On the contrary, it is not possible to count on early detection followed by secondary prevention in those cancer sites where the specific risk factors have not been identified. This is typically the case with lung cancer in which tobacco and occupation hazards represent 90% of the whole risk and in which early detection is very poor and in any case does not ensure a better survival time because of

157

the early metastatic spread of this tumour.

Many sites for which the major risk factors are related to dietary habits can be placed in an intermediate position: this is particularly true for gastro-intestinal cancers. As a matter of fact many doubts still exist on the detailed relationships between diet and these cancers, even though the evidence of an overall relationship of some sort continues to be supported. Indeed we face today a strange situation which is characterized by a continuous increase of knowledge on cancer aetiology and at the same time with a constant increase of cancer mortality. In order to combat this it is important that conclusions on aetiology should be reached. As a matter of urgency, it is essential that more effective and concrete preventive interventions should be planned either of the primary or of the secondary type.

First of all the fight against known risk factors such as tobacco and alcohol must be strongly implemented; these should include educational campaigns and precise and specific legislation.

The approach to other risk factors, such as diet, is more difficult. In this regard two main but contrasting strategies are promoted by researchers: a first group disagree with providing dietary guidelines for the general population at the present while other scientists favour the diffusion of general dietary rules even if we lack conclusive information about the precise relationships between diet and cancer. This problem needs to be considered in a wider context. In particular, it has to be underlined that many pathologies that typically characterize the western countries (i.e. diabetes, cardiovascular diseases, hypertension, overweight and obesity, etc.) are linked with the same diet risk factors which are hypothesized in carcinogenesis.

Therefore, in my opinion, it seems logical to state dietary guidelines and to plan nutritional policies based on claims for a generally healthy diet, and not for a specific cancer prevention diet or for the specific prevention of cardiovascular diseases or diabetes!

In addition to all this, secondary prevention should be strongly supported and favoured, whenever possible.

These short comments suggest the need for European projects dealing with information and education on primary and secondary prevention of cancer, over and above the isolated and national approach. In this regard multiple plans have been developed in the recent years by EEC and in particular by the "Europe against cancer project" and by ECP, as well as by the National Leagues against Cancer.

The general goal foreseen by the "Europe against cancer project" is the 15% decrease of cancer mortality before the year 2000: this result will be fulfilled only if the gap between knowledge and intervention can be overcome.

INDEX OF AUTHORS

SUBJECT INDEX